A Manual of
Oral and Maxillofaci~~~ ~~~g~~y
for Nurses

A Manual of
Oral and Maxillofacial Surgery
for Nurses

Edited by

Colin Yates
BDS, MB, ChB, FDSRCS
Consultant Oral and Maxillofacial Surgeon

**Blackwell
Science**

© 2000 Blackwell Science Ltd
Editorial Offices:
Osney Mead, Oxford OX2 0EL
25 John Street, London WC1N 2BL
23 Ainslie Place, Edinburgh EH3 6AJ
350 Main Street, Malden
  MA 02148 5018, USA
54 University Street, Carlton
  Victoria 3053, Australia
10, rue Casimir Delavigne
  75006 Paris, France

Other Editorial Offices:

Blackwell Wissenschafts-Verlag GmbH
Kurfürstendamm 57
10707 Berlin, Germany

Blackwell Science KK
MG Kodenmacho Building
7-10 Kodenmacho Nihombashi
Chuo-ku, Tokyo 104, Japan

First published 2000

Set in 10/12pt Palatino
by DP Photosetting, Aylesbury, Bucks
Printed and bound in Great Britain by
The Alden Press, Oxford and Northampton

The Blackwell Science logo is a trade mark of
Blackwell Science Ltd, registered at the
United Kingdom Trade Marks Registry

DISTRIBUTORS

Marston Book Services Ltd
PO Box 269
Abingdon
Oxon OX14 4YN
(*Orders:* Tel: 01235 465500
       Fax: 01235 465555)

USA
Blackwell Science, Inc.
Commerce Place
350 Main Street
Malden, MA 02148 5018
(*Orders:* Tel: 800 759 6102
       781 388 8250
       Fax: 781 388 8255)

Canada
Login Brothers Book Company
324 Saulteaux Crescent
Winnipeg, Manitoba R3J 3T2
(*Orders:* Tel: 204 837-2987
       Fax: 204 837-3116)

Australia
Blackwell Science Pty Ltd
54 University Street
Carlton, Victoria 3053
(*Orders:* Tel: 03 9347 0300
       Fax: 03 9347 5001)

A catalogue record for this title is available
from the British Library

ISBN 0-632-05156-6

Library of Congress
Cataloging-in-Publication Data

A manual of oral and maxillofacial surgery
  for nurses/edited by Colin Yates.
     p. ; cm
   Includes bibliographical references and
index.
   ISBN 0-632-05156-6 (pb : alk. paper)
   1. Mouth—Surgery—Handbooks,
manuals, etc.   2. Face—Surgery—
Handbooks, manuals, etc.   3. Surgical
nursing—Handbooks, manuals, etc.
I. Yates, Colin
   [DNLM: 1. Oral Surgical Procedures—
Nurses' Instruction.   2. Stomatognathic
Diseases—surgery—Nurses' Instruction.
WU 600 M294 2000]
RD523.M16 2000
610.73'677—dc21   99-059644

For further information on
Blackwell Science, visit our website:
www.blackwell-science.com

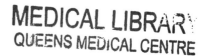

Contents

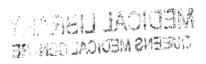

Contributors

Geoffrey T. Cheney RD, FDSRCS, MBBS, LRCP, MRCS, Hon DGDPRCS
Consultant Oral & Maxillofacial Surgeon, Regional Director of Post-graduate Dental Education, Anglia

Peter Cove OStJ, TD, FDSRCS, LRCP, LRCS, FFDRCSI
Consultant Oral & Maxillofacial Surgeon, York District Hospital, York, N. Yorks

Patricia Daymond SRN
Sister, Department of Oral & Maxillofacial Surgery, Wexham Park Hospital, Slough, Berks

Pamela M.D. Edwards SRN
Staff Nurse, Department of Oral & Maxillofacial Surgery, Wexham Park Hospital, Slough, Berks

Richard P. Juniper MBBS, FDSRCS
Honorary Consultant Oral & Maxillofacial Surgeon, John Radcliffe Hospital, Oxford. Regional Director of Postgraduate Dental Education, Oxford

Linda Knighton RGN, Dip NSt
Head & Neck MacMillan Nurse Specialist, Wexham Park Hospital, Slough, Berks

Peter J. Leopard BDS, MBBS, FDSRCS, FRCS(Ed)
Consultant Oral & Maxillofacial Surgeon, North Staffs Hospital, Stoke-on-Trent, Staffs

Gerard Pell BA(Hons), BDS, FDSRCS, MBBS, MRCS, LRCP, Dip Mus
Consultant Oral & Maxillofacial Surgeon, Frenchay Hospital, Bristol, Avon

Clare R. Roberts BDS
Senior House Officer in Oral & Maxillofacial Surgery, Leeds General Infirmary, Leeds, Yorks

G. David D. Roberts MBChB, FDSRCS
Consultant Oral & Maxillofacial Surgeon, York District Hospital, York, N. Yorks

Margot Russell BN, RGN, MSc
Lecturer/Practitioner, Wolfson Institute of Health Science, Thames Valley University

Marianne R.I. Slater RGN
Team Leader, Theatres, Wexham Park Hospital, Slough, Berks

T. John Storrs BDS(Hons), MBBS, FDSRCS
Consultant Oral & Maxillofacial Surgeon, Kent & Canterbury Hospital, Canterbury, Kent

Martin D. Telfer BDS, FDSRCS, MBBS, FRCS
Consultant Oral & Maxillofacial Surgeon, York District Hospital, York, N. Yorks

Colin Yates BDS, MBChB, FDSRCS
Consultant Oral & Maxillofacial Surgeon, Wexham Park Hospital, Slough, Berks

Medical illustrator

Jane Fallows FIMI

Preface

The specialty of oral and maxillofacial surgery deals with diseases, disorders and injuries of the mouth, jaws and face, and is represented in most district general hospitals. It is unique in the surgical specialties in that its senior staff are both dentally and medically qualified, as well as widely trained in dentistry and general and specialist surgery.

The stimulus for this book came from requests from nursing staff on the ward, in the out-patient department and operating theatre, for more information on the various aspects of nursing care related to the specialty. Perusal of the nursing literature reveals a singular lack of relevant written material specifically for nurses.

There are five sections written by nurses working in the out-patient clinics, the ward and the operating theatre, which assume familiarity with general nursing principles and duties. Emphasis is therefore on those aspects relevant to the specialty. The remainder of the book is divided into chapters describing the majority of the conditions and procedures which would be encountered in most units. Some highly specialised topics practised at relatively few centres have been omitted, notably craniofacial surgery, skull base access surgery and primary surgery for cleft lip and palate. In addition, there has been no attempt at comprehensive coverage of 'oral medicine' – the diagnosis and management, often non-surgically, of diseases of the oral mucosa and facial pain.

The nurse's role as patient educator means that he/she must have a clear understanding of why a particular course of action is being taken. Conditions and procedures are therefore covered in terms of relevant background, anatomy and pathology as well as details of pre-operative and post-operative care. Similarly operative procedures are described in some detail with the aim of promoting a deeper understanding of operative technique which will contribute not only to the nurse's traditional role as scrub nurse, but also on occasions as surgical assistant.

Shorter hospital stays with an emphasis on out-patient and day stay surgery make patient information especially important. Examples are given throughout the book as appropriate.

C. Yates

Acknowledgements

In a multi-author text it is difficult to acknowledge adequately the assistance we have all received from many colleagues and from family. Each contributor undoubtedly has several individuals to whom they are indebted for advice and encouragement. We are most grateful to them all.

As editor, however, I must single out my nursing colleagues at Wexham Park Hopital in Slough, our medical illustration department for photographs of the instrument layouts, and my wife, Jenny, for her support, patience and production of the manuscript and index.

Introduction

This series of anatomical diagrams shows the main features of the facial skeleton, the main sensory nerve of the face and mouth (Vth cranial or trigeminal) and the motor nerve for the muscles of facial expression (VIIth cranial or facial). The nomenclature for the teeth is also shown.

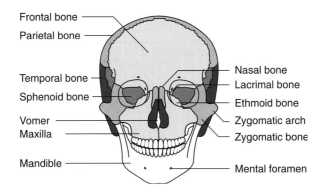

Fig. A   The bones of the skull and facial skeleton.

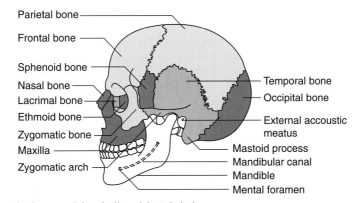

Fig. B   The bones of the skull and facial skeleton.

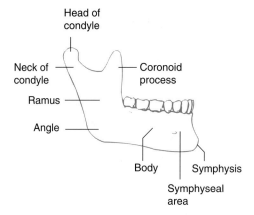

Fig. C   The mandible is divided into regions for descriptive purposes.

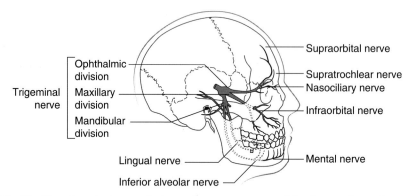

Fig. D   The trigeminal nerve is the main sensory nerve of the face and mouth.

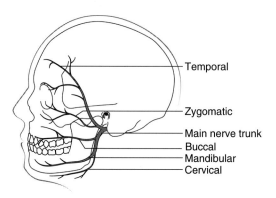

Fig. E   The facial nerve and its branches.

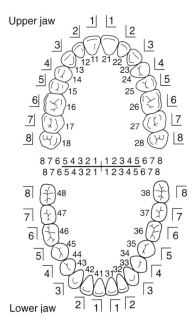

Upper jaw

Lower jaw

Fig. F   The dental formulae. The quadrant system is shown outside the arches, the two-digit system within the arches.

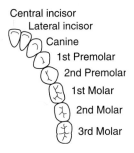

Central incisor
Lateral incisor
Canine
1st Premolar
2nd Premolar
1st Molar
2nd Molar
3rd Molar

Fig. G   The teeth by name.

1

The Out-patient Department

P. Daymond

This chapter describes the role of the nurse in the organisation and running of the out-patient department.

Communication with patients

Nurses should be aware that the patient's visit to the out-patient clinic may be their first contact with the hospital and it is especially important to ensure that they are treated with the maximum care and consideration.

The department should be kept neat and tidy at all times and nurses should be observant of patients' needs, particularly with regard to the elderly and frail. It is useful to have a good supply of magazines in the waiting area to keep patients occupied whilst they are waiting for their appointment. Some children's books are also essential, as well as a few toys for the younger visitors.

It should be noted that according to the Patient's Charter (DOH 1995) the waiting time should not exceed 30 minutes. A notice board, which can be updated, to keep patients informed of any delays that are likely to occur can save a lot of frustration for both them and the staff. Information leaflets are also a considerable help in promoting good communication with the patients (*see* Information leaflets Nos 1, 2 and 5 and those in appropriate sections).

It is necessary for the nurse to be skilled in all the aspects of the department, including dealing with emergencies, and all minor treatments and surgery carried out under local anaesthetic. Good communication skills are also required when talking to patients and liaising with medical staff and other departments within the hospital.

The receptionist

The receptionist is a very important person in aiding the smooth running of clinics, and is responsible for collecting notes, X-rays, pathology reports, etc. The nurse must do her best to provide as much information as possible about emergencies and any extra patients who are to be seen during the clinic. On arrival it is essential that the receptionist checks that all the details are correct on the patient's record card and on the computer, before passing the notes onto the clinic nurse.

New patient and follow-up clinics

With the exception of some emergency patients, the out-patient department will be the route by which almost all patients enter care in the specialty.

Clinics may be:

- Diagnostic
- Treatment
- Follow-up

PATIENT INFORMATION LEAFLET No 1

ORAL and MAXILLOFACIAL SURGERY DEPARTMENT

MINOR ORAL SURGERY OPERATIONS
(LOCAL ANAESTHETIC)

1. After your initial consultation with the doctor your name will be placed on the local anaesthetic waiting list. An appointment will be sent to you when your name reaches the top of the list.
2. On the day of your operation please report to the department at the appointed time. There is no need to starve before your appointment – please eat normally.
3. You will be given a local anaesthetic (an injection into the gum) which freezes the area so that you will not feel any pain during the operation. The numbness will take about $1\frac{1}{2}$ to 2 hours to wear off. Be careful not to bite or burn yourself whilst your mouth is still numb.
4. After surgery of the mouth or jaws some swelling and discomfort is not abnormal.
5. You may need to take pain killers such as paracetamol. An antibiotic may also be prescribed.
6. Keeping your mouth clean is important and further instructions will be given to you following the surgery.
7. You may have some stitches but these will usually fall out themselves and can take up to 3 weeks to do so.
8. You should be fit to drive home, but if you feel you would be happier, please bring an escort.
9. You may eat and drink anything you feel you can manage following the operation, usually fairly soft food on the day, taking a normal diet when you feel able. Do not drink anything too hot or too cold for the first few hours.
10. You will usually be given a follow-up appointment.
11. If you need to change your operation appointment, please ring
    . . . .

PATIENT INFORMATION LEAFLET No 2

ORAL and MAXILLOFACIAL SURGERY DEPARTMENT

POST-OPERATIVE INSTRUCTIONS

1. After surgery of the mouth or jaws some swelling and discomfort is not abnormal. An ice pack such as a bag of frozen peas can help to reduce this and may also be very soothing.
2. Slight oozing and blood staining of your saliva for several hours is not unusual.
3. Avoid very hot, hard or chewy foods on the same day as the procedure.
4. You may need to take painkillers such as paracetamol or ibuprofen. An antibiotic may also be prescribed.
5. It is important to keep your mouth clean and you should brush as normally as possible, but in the wound area use a mouth rinse, e.g. hot salt water, hot solution of bicarbonate or a mouth wash, three or four times a day starting the following day, until you are able to brush normally.
6. You may have some stitches but these will usually fall out themselves.
7. You will usually be given a follow-up appointment.
8. If you have special problems following the operation, ring . . . . for advice.

Diagnosis will normally be achieved at the first visit and include any investigations which are necessary (e.g. X-ray). Following diagnosis, patients are directed as appropriate for treatment (if necessary) and follow up. New and follow-up patients are often seen in the same clinics. Treatment is normally carried out in specially designated clinics.

The clinic must be prepared and equipped with disposables and instruments according to the preferences of the clinician, but for routine examination would include:

- Dental mirrors and probes
- Instruments for suture removal (both intra- and extra-oral)
- Headlight if required

In addition, adequate supplies of all necessary stationery must be readily available, especially the most commonly used request forms:

- X-ray/imaging
- Pathology
- Waiting list

The patient is then called into the clinic, and greeted politely by the nurse in charge. After the consultation and examination by the doctor, the patient may be asked to go to the X-ray department before a diagnosis can be made or a decision taken on treatment. Once returned from X-ray the patient may well be invited to see the doctor again for a further discussion on the findings. If the patient requires an operation, a waiting list card is completed by the doctor and these details will be added to the patient's existing computerised records, and the patient given the appropriate information sheet. It is very important to ensure that full details are entered on the card, especially contact telephone numbers.

Emergency patients

A proportion of emergency patients will enter care via the out-patient department. They should be seen and assessed as soon as possible. Treatment may be carried out in the out-patient clinic or admission arranged to the ward if necessary.

Treatment clinics

Minor oral surgery

The decision to carry out surgical treatment under local anaesthetic in the out-patient department, as opposed to admission for surgery under general anaesthesia on a day stay basis is based on several factors. These are:

- Surgical complexity and length of procedure
- Age, medical and social status of the patient
- The patient's preference

In the specialty, a large volume of minor and intermediate surgical work is carried out on an out-patient basis in the minor oral surgery (MOS) clinic including dental extractions, surgical extractions, apicectomy, biopsy and soft tissue surgery and cryotherapy. In addition, emergency treatment such as drainage of abscesses, and the repair of lacerations will be undertaken.

Trolleys are washed down with detergent and water and dried, then sprayed with 70% alcohol. The appropriate instruments are assembled for the procedure to be undertaken, including three basic surgical trays (*see also* Chapter 4):

■ Surgical tray No 1 (*see* Fig. 4.5), which is comprehensive and may be modified according to preference and the procedure to be undertaken
■ Surgical tray No 2 (*see* Fig. 4.6), which is specifically for periapical surgery
■ Surgical tray No 3 (*see* Fig. 4.7), which is for soft tissue surgery and biopsy
■ A selection of dental extraction forceps (*see* Fig. 4.8)

In addition the following items of equipment and disposable accessories must be prepared:

■ Suction unit – suction connection tubing and disposable bags
■ Drill unit with irrigation, surgical handpieces and burs
■ Dental syringes and local anaesthetic
■ Sutures
■ Disposable plastic covers for the dental chair controls and light
■ Gloves, gowns and masks for the surgeon and assistant
■ Bib and protective goggles or spectacles for the patient
■ Sterile drapes as required

It is very important for the nursing staff to understand and appreciate the great stress and fear that some patients undergoing surgery under local anaesthetic are experiencing when they attend the clinic. Every effort must be made to relax the patient and a knowledge of some simple relaxation techniques may be helpful. Gentle music playing softly in the background can assist in relieving tension. Some individuals find it comforting to hold the nurse's hand whilst receiving the local anaesthetic injection. It may also be helpful to provide the patient with a relaxation information sheet when they are put on the waiting list at their first visit so that they can practise some of the techniques before attending for a procedure (Information leaflet No 3).

■ After the patient has been shown into the treatment room and their personal details checked, they are asked to sign a consent form and the surgeon makes sure that they understand the procedure to be carried out. The doctor will also check the patient's current medication and medical history. If the patient has mistakenly missed a meal prior to coming to the hospital, it is advisable to give a glucose drink before

PATIENT INFORMATION LEAFLET No 3

ORAL and MAXILLOFACIAL DEPARTMENT

RELAXATION INFORMATION SHEET

Most people find a visit to the dentist very stressful and relaxation exercises might be quite helpful in making you feel more at ease before your appointment.

Preparation for relaxation
Sit or lie quietly in a comfortable room. If sitting, take off your shoes, uncross your legs and rest your arms on the arms of the chair. If lying, lie on your back with your arms at your sides. Close your eyes and become aware of your body. Notice how you are breathing. Ensure you are comfortable. Here are a few techniques which might help you to relax. They are easy to perform, but require practice.

Techniques for relieving physical tension
Imagine that you are wearing a jacket over a shirt, the sleeve of which has got caught and you cannot reach it so try to shake it down. Shake one arm two or three times, repeat with the other arm.

Body stretching helps over-tensed muscles to relax. To relieve tension in the hands, open the fingers to stretch the muscles on the palms. Then relax.

To relieve shoulder tension, stretch the top of the head upwards, drop the shoulders. There is then a recoil which produces a relaxed feeling.

Other muscles may be stretched to relieve tension, but this should not cause pain.

Body scanning technique. This means that you can mentally look at your body, either starting from the feet and working up, or from the head and working down, spotting any points of tension which you can relax by alternately tensing and relaxing the muscles concerned.

Affirmation technique. Which means that you talk to yourself. You develop short phrases which you can say to yourself when feeling tense, e.g. 'I feel relaxed' or 'Stop worrying'.

►

PATIENT INFORMATION LEAFLET No 3 *continued*

Visualisation. This means that you develop a picture in your mind of a favourite place where you have spent a happy time, or just let your imagination take you on a journey. For example, imagine you are walking on a beach with the warm golden sand between your toes and your feet sinking into the sand as you walk. You can feel the warm sunshine on your skin and there is a slight breeze from the sea. You are watching the waves flowing towards the shore and gently breaking on the sand.

Breathing awareness. First let the air out of your lungs as slowly as you can. Do not force it. Now breathe in slowly, but not deeply, and let your breathing settle into its natural pattern. As your breathing settles think of the expansion in the lower part of your chest. You can do this by placing your hand on your stomach. Continue to breathe evenly and gently.

Other useful exercises
- Curl your toes and press your feet down
- Press your heels down and bend your feet up
- Tense your calf muscles
- Tense your thigh muscles
- Make your buttocks tight
- Tense your stomach as if to receive a punch
- Bend your elbows and tense the muscles of your arms
- Hunch your shoulders and press your head back into the cushion or pillow
- Clench your jaws, frown and screw up your eyes really tight
- Tense all of your muscles together
- Do each of the above for 10 seconds, then relax
- Close your eyes
- Focus your mind on an imaginary white rose against a black background for 30 seconds as you breathe slowly and quietly
- Open your eyes

Conclusion
Practice is very important if you are going to gain any benefit from any of the above techniques. It is no good waiting until you are stressed and tense before you try them. As you become more practised you will be able to do on the spot relaxation at times of stress. If you are relaxed you will find a visit to the dentist less traumatic.

commencing any procedure as this will help to prevent the patient from fainting.

■ The patient is then asked to sit in the dental chair and made as comfortable as possible. A bib is placed around the neck and goggles worn to protect the eyes from any instruments passed across the face, or water splashes. Every effort must be made to make the patient comfortable and relaxed, which is not an easy task as most patients are extremely nervous at the prospect of surgical treatment.

■ After scrubbing, the surgeon puts on gown and gloves. The local anaesthetic is given after it has first been checked by both the doctor and nurse. The nurse then prepares to assist, by scrubbing up and donning sterile gown/apron and gloves.

■ During the operation it is important for the assistant to keep the operation site clear of any blood, water or saliva and retract efficiently so that the surgeon can see the operating field clearly at all times. It is also important to ensure that the patient's condition remains stable. Patients in the dental chair are prone to faint, so it is necessary to be observant and notice any change of colour, sweating or agitation.

■ When the procedure is completed, the bib is removed and the patient's face is cleaned if necessary. When feeling well enough, the patient is invited to leave the dental chair to sit by the surgeon who will give post-operative instructions and a prescription for any drugs which may be necessary. A written post-operative instruction sheet will also be given to the patient as well as an appointment for a post-operative review.

■ After the procedure all instruments are carefully washed and dried and replaced in instrument trays ready for sterilisation. The trolley is washed down with water and detergent, dried, and sprayed with 70% alcohol. The dental chair is similarly treated between procedures and spittoons are cleaned and rinsed before the next patient is brought into the room.

■ At the end of the session, chair, spittoon and all surfaces are recleaned as before, and waste filter and aspirating tubes are flushed through with non-foaming antibacterial fluid. The suction trap is cleaned and disinfected. The spittoon is also rinsed through with an antibacterial solution.

Intravenous sedation

■ Most departments will have their own protocol for patients having treatment under sedation. Detailed information sheets are essential and an example is provided (Information leaflet No 4)

■ Equipment should be ready before the patient comes into the treatment room since any delay can increase the patient's anxiety:
  □ Tourniquet
  □ Mediswabs

PATIENT INFORMATION LEAFLET No 4

ORAL and MAXILLOFACIAL SURGERY DEPARTMENT

INTRAVENOUS SEDATION

You will be given INTRAVENOUS SEDATION for your treatment. This has been explained to you. In your own interest, please follow these instructions to protect yourself and avoid accidents.

ON THE DAY OF TREATMENT

DO bring a responsible adult with you who is able to wait and escort you home. Sedation will NOT be given if you arrive without an escort.

DO have a light meal before treatment at least 4 hours before your appointment.

DON'T eat fatty foods or drink any alcohol.

DURING THE 24 HOURS FOLLOWING TREATMENT

DO travel home with your escort, by car if possible.

DO stay resting quietly at home for the rest of the day.

DON'T drive for 24 hours.

DON'T use complex machinery (e.g. cookers, washing machines, power tools).

DON'T sign any important legal or business documents.

DON'T drink any alcohol.

If you have any queries at all, please call us on . . . .

- ☐ Butterfly/intravenous cannula
- ☐ Adhesive tape
- ☐ Pulse oximeter
- ☐ Sphygmomanometer
- ☐ Oxygen supply and Ventimask
- ☐ Drugs, e.g.
  - – Midazolam
  - – Flumazenil
- ☐ Syringes and needles

- The patient is invited into the treatment room and made comfortable, and the consent form completed.
- The pulse oximeter probe is applied and checked that it is recording correctly.
- The sphygmomanometer cuff is applied on the opposite arm to the intravenous site.
- The intravenous cannula is inserted and secured with adhesive tape.
- The drug is checked and administered and the amount given recorded in the patient's notes.
- When the patient is adequately sedated, local anaesthetic is given and the procedure is carried out.
- Oxygen saturation and pulse rate are monitored continuously throughout the procedure.
- On completion of the procedure the patient is moved to the recovery area for observation.
- The intravenous cannula is removed when the patient's condition is satisfactory.
- When fully recovered the patient is discharged by the surgeon with appropriate written post-operative instructions.

Dental impressions

Impressions of the mouth and teeth are taken in the clinic in relation to a variety of conditions:

- To construct splints for the support of loosened or dislodged teeth
- To construct splints for the treatment of temporo-mandibular joint problems
- To construct study models and splints for the assessment and treatment of patients undergoing orthognathic surgery
- To construct prostheses for patients following surgery for jaw and facial cancer

Materials and equipment required for taking impressions:

- Bib for patient
- Impression trays and fixative

- Alginate impression material and measure
- Measure for water
- Mixing bowl and spatula
- Labels and laboratory forms
- Antibacterial rinse for impression, wet gauze and plastic bag

The procedure is as follows:

- The patient sits in the dental chair with the head well supported
- An impression tray is selected and checked for size
- Fixative may be applied to the tray
- The impression material is mixed and applied to the tray and placed in the patient's mouth
- After the impression material has set, the tray is removed and the impression checked for accuracy
- The impression is rinsed in an antibacterial solution, labelled, covered with damp gauze and placed in an airtight polythene bag
- A laboratory card is completed and the impression delivered to the laboratory without delay

Summary

The nurse's role in the out-patient clinic is:

- To ensure that clinics run smoothly and efficiently
- To ensure that patients are given the necessary care and attention when attending clinics
- To be responsible for the sterilisation, care and maintenance of equipment

Good communication skills are essential.

2

Pre-assessment

P. Edwards

This chapter describes the role of the nurse in the organisation and running of pre-assessment clinics.

Role of the pre-assessment nurse

- To effectively manage and monitor specialty pre-assessment clinics and waiting lists, liaising with all disciplines to co-ordinate a quality service to patients before admission.
- To undertake an assessment of all patients prior to admission, and provide patients and relatives with information regarding condition, admission and outcome.
- To assess which patients, e.g. those for cancer or orthognathic surgery, and their relatives will require more time for a detailed discussion of all aspects of their forthcoming treatment.
- To plan and arrange operating lists, ensuring the effective utilisation of operating time.
- To manage the waiting list according to hospital policy and guidelines.
- To deal with waiting list enquiries.

Reasons for pre-assessment

- To check that patients are fit to undergo an operation, usually under general anaesthetic.
- To enable existing medical problems to be stabilised prior to surgery.
- To organise any procedures that are required prior to surgery.
- To ensure that all relevant paperwork is completed prior to surgery.
- To allocate patients to the most suitable ward e.g. day surgery unit (Fig. 2.1), 5-day ward, or main ward.
- To inform patients and their relatives about the operation, hospital stay and after-care.

Day Surgery Unit

ADMISSION CRITERIA FOR SURGERY UNDER GENERAL ANAESTHETIC

Ideally patients should be ASA I or II. However, the decision to operate must be made after an overall consideration of the nature of the planned operation, together with the general medical fitness of the patient. Consideration should also include the following:

AGE   Physiological age may be more relevant than age in years
       Children <16 years must be on designated paediatric lists

STATURE   Height and weight are measured to allow calculation of body mass index (BMI, or Quetelet value). An upper limit of approximately 30 is generally agreed

SOCIAL   Can get to DSU by 08:00 – escort home by 18:00
          Adult supervision at home post op for 24 hours

GENERAL   Ambulant
Can adequately self-administer post-operative analgesia
Clinically and psychologically fit

PRE-OPERATIVE INVESTIGATIONS
Haemoglobin where indicated – should be >10g/dl
Sickle test where appropriate
MRSA screening if appropriate

EXCLUDE PATIENTS WITH

CARDIOVASCULAR DISEASE	**Unstable** angina Heart failure Heart block or dysrhythmia **Recent** myocardial infarction or CVA Hypertension **(systolic less than 160 mmHg, diastolic less than 100 mmHg)**
RESPIRATORY DISEASE	Acute respiratory infections Severe asthma, e.g. if requiring systemic steroids Chronic obstructive airways disease, if unable to climb 1 flight of stairs
METABOLIC etc.	Alcoholism, narcotic addiction Diabetes – **insulin dependent** Renal failure, liver disease Haemophilia
NEURO MUSCULO SKELETAL	Arthritis of jaw, neck, or hip Cervical spondylosis Myasthenia, myopathies, etc. Multiple sclerosis
DRUGS	Steroids, MAOIs Anticoagulants Antidysrhythmics, e.g. Verapamil

If in doubt please telephone the Senior Nurse, Day Surgery Unit
Communication is everything

Fig. 2.1   Admission criteria for day surgery under general anaesthetic.

■ To arrange suitable operation dates for patients and allow them to organise their work and domestic commitments so that their operation causes least disruption.
■ To organise efficient operating lists which fully utilise operating theatre time.
■ To reduce failure to attend on the day of operation and therefore to reduce waiting list time.

The pre-assessment clinic

A suitable examination room is required with equipment and facilities for the nurse and doctor to carry out the pre-assessment procedure. All current notes and X-rays for patients attending the clinic must be available.

The pre-assessment nurse

- The patient is asked to fill in a health questionnaire (Fig. 2.2).
- Personal details are taken (Figs 2.3 & 2.4).
- Routine observations are recorded:
  - □ blood pressure
  - □ pulse
  - □ respiration
  - □ weight and height are recorded to allow calculation of the body mass index (BMI, Quetelet index)
  - □ urine analysis

Information given to patients

The pre-assessment nurse gives patients the following information:

- Date and time of operation
- Time for nil by mouth and reasons
- Whether current medication needs to be taken prior to the operation and at what time it should be taken
- Time to arrive on the ward
- What to bring to the hospital (clothing, toiletries and current medication, e.g. inhalers)
- Details of transfer to the operating theatre
- Immediate effects of surgery and general anaesthetic (Information leaflet No 5)
- Discharge procedure including:
  - □ drugs to take out
  - □ post-operative wound/mouth care
  - □ recovery period and time off work
  - □ follow-up appointment
- Contact telephone numbers if there are any problems
- Information regarding the possibility of the operation date being cancelled due to emergency cases
- Specific information relating to day surgery (Figs 2.5 and 2.6)
- Verbal information is reinforced by written information sheets relating to the type of surgery and length of stay

DETAILS OF PAST MEDICAL HISTORY AND GENERAL HEALTH

To be completed by patient when possible.

Have you had any operations in the past?   YES/NO

If yes, what were they for?

Did you have a   If yes, did you have any adverse reactions?
general anaesthetic?

(Please answer the following questions if they are appropriate to you by circling YES or NO and add details where required)

1. Are you allergic to anything?   YES NO
   Please specify . . . .
2. Do you bring up phlegm from
   your chest?   YES NO
3. Have you had a cold/sore throat
   in the last 3 weeks?   YES NO
4. Does your chest ever sound
   wheezy?   YES NO
5. Do your ankles swell most days? YES NO
6. Do you get more short of breath
   than other people your own age:
   a. when climbing hills/stairs?   YES NO
   b. walking on level ground?   YES NO
7. Do you have any bowel
   problems?   YES NO
8. Have you ever had pain or
   discomfort in your chest:
   a. when you exercise or hurry?   YES NO
   b. does it disappear on resting? YES NO
9. Are you or your parents of African
   or Eastern Mediterranean origin? YES NO
   If yes, have you had a Sickle
   Cell test?   YES NO
10. Have you or any member of your
    family had a problem with an
    anaesthetic?   YES NO
11. Do you have any loose/capped/
    crowned or false teeth?   YES NO

Have you had or do you suffer from:
12. Tuberculosis   YES NO
13. Heart trouble (pain/palpitations)   YES NO
14. Rheumatic fever   YES NO
15. High blood pressure   YES NO
16. Chest trouble/asthma   YES NO
17. Liver disease/jaundice   YES NO
18. Kidney disease   YES NO
19. Diabetes   YES NO
20. Thyroid disorders   YES NO
21. Bruising or bleeding tendencies   YES NO
22. Thrombosis (blood clots)   YES NO
23. Severe anxiety/depression   YES NO
24. A stroke   YES NO
25. Epilepsy/convulsions/fits   YES NO
26. Dizzy spells   YES NO
27. Sciatica or back trouble   YES NO
28. Neck or jaw trouble   YES NO
29. Heartburn/indigestion/hiatus
    hernia   YES NO
30. Do you smoke? (How many?)   YES NO

31. Do you drink alcohol?
    (How much?) . . . . YES NO
32. Are you pregnant?   YES NO
33. Are there any other medical
    problems?   YES NO
    List below please.

Write further details of medical problems here.

Fig. 2.2   Details of past medical history and general health.

NURSE CLERKING ASSESSMENT FORM

NAME	HOSPITAL No	MALE/FEMALE
ADDRESS	D.o.B.	AGE
	RELIGION	OCCUPATION
POST CODE TEL No HOME WORK	WHAT WOULD YOU LIKE TO BE CALLED?	ETHNIC ORIGIN

CONSULTANT	DATE OF ADMISSION
T.C.I. DATE	PRE-ASSESSED BY
PLANNED DISCHARGE DATE	DATE
ACTUAL DISCHARGE DATE	NAMED NURSE
REASON FOR ANY DELAY	WARD

NEXT OF KIN ADDRESS	GP ADDRESS
TEL No & WORK No RELATIONSHIP INFORMED OF ADMISSION? YES/NO 2nd CONTACT: NAME RELATIONSHIP TEL No	MEDICATION TAKEN OVER LAST 4 WEEKS ALLERGIES

SOURCE OF ADMISSION(✓)   CLINIC   PLANNED   A&E   GP

PAST MEDICAL HISTORY (MAJOR DIAGNOSTIC LABELS ONLY e.g. 'DIABETES')

REASON FOR ADMISSION – INCLUDE PATIENT'S EXPLANATION

OPERATION TO BE PERFORMED & DATE

Fig. 2.3   Nurse clerking assessment form.

Section A. SOCIAL SUPPORT

ACCOMMODATION: House / Flat / Bungalow / Lodgings / Residential Care / Nursing Home

Warden-controlled?   Alarm System?
Toilet: Upstairs / Downstairs / Both
Bathroom: Upstairs / Downstairs / Both
Will the patient have to climb stairs at home?
Lives alone / With spouse / Relatives / Other

DEPENDANTS: Spouse / Children / Other
Who is caring for this person in the patient's absence

INFORMAL CARER: Name: Relationship:
Address: Nature of help:

Tel No   Can this continue?
Has this been confirmed by carer?

OTHER USEFUL INFORMATION:

Section B: COMMUNITY SUPPORT

GP: Address:

Health / Social Services:

| | On Admission | | | On Discharge | | |
	How Often	Aware of Admission	Needed	How Often	Arranged	Start Date
District Nurse						
Health Visitor						
Home Care/Help						
MOW						
Day Centre						
Community SW						
Community OT						
Other						

Section C: MULTIDISCIPLINARY TEAM

	Date Referred	Date Referred	Arranged
Physio			
O.T.			
Speech Therapy			
Dietitian			
Social Worker			
Other			

Fig. 2.4   Social and community support.

PATIENT INFORMATION LEAFLET No 5

ORAL and MAXILLOFACIAL SURGERY DEPARTMENT

INSTRUCTIONS FOR PATIENTS AFTER A GENERAL ANAESTHETIC

Some anaesthetic drugs remain in the body for 24 to 48 hours and during this time are gradually excreted. During this period you are under the influence of drugs and should not do certain things.

DON'T   Drive a car or any form of motorised transport, or bicycles.

DON'T   Drink alcohol.

DON'T   Operate any machinery or electrical appliances, including a kettle or saucepan.

DON'T   Make important decisions.

DON'T   Lock the bathroom or toilet door or in any way make yourself inaccessible to the person looking after you.

DON'T   Watch too much TV or read too much as this may cause blurred vision.

DO   Drink plenty of fluids, but avoid hot drinks and food for 24 hours as this may cause bleeding. Tepid or lukewarm food and drink should be taken, but not too much tea or coffee. A light diet should be taken, but nothing very heavy or greasy as this could result in nausea.

DO   Rest quietly at home on the day of discharge. It may take 2 to 3 days before the weariness wears off and occasional lapses of concentration may occur for up to a week after the operation.

Anaesthetic drugs may cause flu-like symptoms in the following days and there may be aching joints or generalised muscular pains. A sore throat or blocked nose (due to the tube passed during operation) may be treated with paracetamol or ibuprofen.

If any problems develop which fail to respond to the treatment outlined, please phone . . . .

ESCORT INFORMATION

TO THE ESCORT OF:

NAME. . . . .

Please collect the patient at . . . . am/pm from the Day Surgery Unit

PLEASE READ THE FOLLOWING INSTRUCTIONS CAREFULLY

The patient must be taken home in a private care and kept under supervision for at least 24 hours.

You are reminded that the patient must not be allowed to drive a car or any other vehicle, or to operate apparatus or machinery (including cookers) for 24 hours after discharge from the Day Surgery Unit.

Please leave your telephone number with the Receptionist so that we may contact you should the need arise.

Yours faithfully

SISTER IN CHARGE

Fig. 2.5   Escort information.

Children and teenagers attend a normal pre-assessment clinic and are then invited to visit the paediatric ward so that they can see the ward and meet the nurses/playleaders who will be involved in their care. This is actively encouraged at the pre-assessment session and the relevant information given to the parent or guardian (Information leaflet No 6).

The doctor

■ The patient's completed health questionnaire is checked.
■ A physical examination is performed and details recorded.
■ The operation/procedure is explained.
■ Time is allowed for the patient (parent/guardian) to ask questions.
■ The consent form is signed.
■ The patient may be sent for any relevant pre-operative investigations (Fig. 2.7).
■ If the patient is found to be medically unfit at pre-assessment they will referred to their general medical practitioner or appropriate consultant, for management. The patient will be re-assessed once stabilised.
■ Patients with complex medical histories will be referred to the consultant anaesthetist for assessment.

DAY SURGERY UNIT

THE DATE FOR YOUR OPERATION ON THE DAY SURGERY UNIT IS . . . .

PLEASE NOTE: ANY FAILURE TO ATTEND FOR THE OPERATION WITHOUT NOTIFYING THE DAY SURGERY UNIT WILL RESULT IN YOUR REMOVAL FROM THE WAITING LIST.

Unless the following conditions are fulfilled, it will not be possible to carry our your operation.

A) **YOU SHOULD ARRIVE AT THE DAY SURGERY UNIT AT** . . . . **THERE IS NO NEED TO PHONE FOR A BED.**

B) **NO FOOD OR DRINK MUST BE TAKEN FROM MIDNIGHT.**

LIGHT EARLY BREAKFAST BEFORE 8.00 AM (E.G. TOAST, CEREAL, TEA OR COFFEE). NOTHING AT ALL AFTER 8.00 AM.

c) Arrangements are made by you to be taken home in a car or taxi by a responsible adult (you will not be allowed home on your own).

d) You undertake that there will be someone at home to look after you for at least 24 hours after you return home.

e) You undertake not to drive a car or any other vehicle or cycle or to operate apparatus or machinery (including cookers) for 24 hours after your return home.

f) You are particularly asked NOT to wear watches or jewellery (other than wedding rings) or to bring large sums of money or valuables to the Unit on the day of your admission. You may need change for the telephone.

g) DO NOT work the night before your operation.

h) Your wash things are not required, but please bring in your dressing gown.

i) DO NOT wear any make-up or nail varnish. Please leave your handbag at home.

j) Please wear flat shoes.

k) Please have a bath before admission.

l) Please bring your medical card with you.

m) Enquire prior to admission if you should continue to take regular medication and bring any medication or inhalers you are using.

If after you have accepted this appointment date you find that you are unable to keep it please telephone the Unit on . . . . **to make another appointment. Please notify us if you have suffered from any acute illness such as a cold or sore throat in the 2 weeks prior to the operation.**

Day Surgery is a mixed sex ward. Please note that the Hospital operates a No Smoking Policy.

The staff of the Day Surgery Unit wish to make your stay and treatment as comfortable as possible. Please telephone the unit if you have any problems.

Fig. 2.6   Day Surgery Unit instructions.

RECOMMENDATIONS FOR PRE-OPERATIVE INVESTIGATIONS OF PATIENTS FOR ELECTIVE SURGERY

CHEST RADIOGRAPH
1. Cardiorespiratory disease
2. Possible pulmonary malignancy (Primary or secondary)
3. Severe trauma
4. Immigrants from countries with endemic TB (1 and 4 – if no radiograph within the last 12 months)

ELECTROCARDIOGRAPH
1. Patients older than 60 years undergoing major surgery
2. Symptoms and signs of cardiovascular disease, including ischaemic heart disease or hypertension
3. Symptomatic respiratory disease

UREA AND ELECTROLYTES
1. Clinical evidence of renal disease
2. Symptomatic cardiovascular disease
3. Diabetes
4. Drugs – diuretics, digoxin, steroids, others causing electrolyte disturbances

LIVER FUNCTION TESTS
1. Clinical evidence of liver disease
2. Chronic liver disease, including a history of hepatitis

FULL BLOOD COUNT
1. Major surgery
2. Chronic bleeding
3. History of anaemia
4. Renal disease

CLOTTING SCREEN
1. Clinical evidence of liver disease including a history of hepatitis
2. Bleeding disorder
3. Anticoagulants
4. Renal disease

MISCELLANEOUS

CXR	. . . .	× Match	. . . .
ECG	. . . .	Group & save	. . . .
Abdo X-ray	. . . .	How many:	. . . .
Ultrasound	. . . .	Hold serum only	. . . .
IVP	. . . .	FBC	. . . .
CT	. . . .	ESR	. . . .
U & Es	. . . .	INR	. . . .
LFTs	. . . .	APPT	. . . .
Glucose	. . . .	Sickle	. . . .
Audio	. . . .	Photography	. . . .
Laser	. . . .		

Fig. 2.7 Recommendations for pre-operative investigations for elective surgery.

PATIENT INFORMATION LEAFLET No 6

ORAL and MAXILLOFACIAL SURGERY DEPARTMENT

CHILDREN

Information for parents/guardians

The Children's Ward like all children and teenagers to visit prior to their surgery, and this visit can be combined with pre-assessment. Information regarding when to visit will be sent to you with the admission letter and operation date (generally about 2 weeks prior to the operation). Please bring your child along as it will allow them to see the ward and the nurses/play leader and information will be given to you about what to expect on the day of the operation. It is helpful that any fears are allayed and all questions answered before the day of operation. This visit will enable you and your child to discuss arrangements with the staff to ensure a stay that is as enjoyable as possible.

Please phone . . . . if your child develops a cough or cold in the week prior to the operation date so that alternative arrangements may be made. Your child may need to be treated by your General Practitioner in the meantime.

You will be told at pre-assessment about when your child has to stop eating and drinking. This depends on what time your child will be going to theatre. It is **very important** to follow these directions carefully as an empty stomach is required prior to surgery. It is necessary to phone on the morning of the operation to ensure the bed is still available. This is an emergency hospital and there are times when surgical beds have been taken by urgent cases. If your child's operation is cancelled on the day of the operation, because there are no beds, another date for operation will be given within 3 to 4 weeks of the original date.

All parents are encouraged to stay with their child for the day and to accompany their child to the anaesthetic room. You will be informed as soon as your child is ready to be collected from the recovery room.

▶

PATIENT INFORMATION LEAFLET No 6 *continued*

Your child will be allowed home after being seen by one of the surgeons and advice given on when he/she may return to school.

For the first 24 hours after the operation your child should be kept quiet and under close supervision. He/she should be encouraged to drink and have a soft diet if necessary. Some of the anaesthetic drugs can cause dizziness and sickness or flu-like symptoms, so plenty of rest and painkillers are recommended, and not too much television or reading. A blocked or stuffy nose can also occur due to a tube being passed during the operation. This will improve after a few days. If there are any stitches they will be dissolvable, and will come out on their own.

We suggest you ensure that you have a supply of suitable painkillers at home e.g. paracetamol. Antibiotics may be provided by the Hospital. Regular oral hygiene (mouthwashes and tooth brushing) also plays an important role in preventing infection and you will be given an instruction sheet on discharge.

A follow-up out-patient appointment will be given for the following week.

If you have any problems following the operation ring . . . . for advice.

Summary

- The pre-assessment clinic (often nurse led) has an essential part to play in the running of any surgical department.
- Pre-assessment of patients is especially relevant to day surgery when the patient's time at hospital is reduced to a minimum.
- The role of the pre-assessment nurse is often extended to the management of waiting lists and the compilation of operating lists.

3

The Ward and Day Unit

M. Russell

This chapter examines the care of patients who require admission to either a ward or day unit for oral and maxillofacial surgery.

Patient selection and admission to hospital

Prior to any admission to hospital, no matter how minor the procedure may be, there is still a certain degree of associated anxiety. Generally this is a fear of the unknown, as hospitals are an alien environment to the majority of the general public. However if it is appreciated that an operation to the head and neck area may not only affect normal every-day functions such as eating, drinking and communicating, but also appearance, the anxiety levels can be expected to increase greatly. As discussed before, pre-operative assessment provides an ideal forum, not only for obtaining information from the patient but also for the alleviation of anxieties by both nursing and medical staff. The provision of adequate and appropriate information pre-operatively reduces anxiety levels and can assist in an uneventful post-operative period as the patient feels more in control of their situation, thus lessening their fear of the unknown.

In the previous chapter, assessment of patients prior to their admission to hospital was discussed. Pre-admission clinics provide a vital service, not just in the reduction of patient anxieties but also in the selection of patients in terms of whether they are suitable to be a day case or require an extended stay in hospital. Day surgery units have strict criteria for admission to the unit. Elderly and frail patients may often be excluded as the potential for complications developing post-operatively is greatly increased. Patients with underlying medical conditions such as epilepsy or those who require anticoagulant therapy may also require admission to a ward rather than a Day Unit due to the risks involved during the post-operative phase of care.

Other factors which should be taken into consideration are time of day of operation, support at home and transport for the return journey. However, clinical judgement must be used when discharging patients from hospital, as sometimes the unexpected will occur and the intended day case patient may require admission to a ward due to unexpected complications from either anaesthesia or surgery. As with any discharge home, the nurse is accountable for ensuring the safety and appropriateness of the patient for discharge.

Nursing process and patient assessment

Although the nursing process may seem 'old hat' as nursing progresses into the millennium, it is imperative in providing a firm base upon which patient care and nursing interventions are planned. It is important to establish what is normal for each individual, in terms of their day to day living, in order to be able to plan the most appropriate care for both the pre-operative and post-operative phases of their hospital experience.

If one examines the process in more detail it can be seen that assessment of patients is only the first step in providing appropriate, evidence based care. The nursing process can be represented schematically:

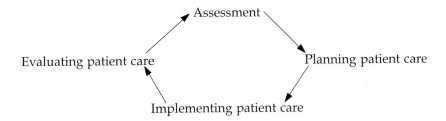

Once a full assessment is made, be it in a pre-admission clinic or on a ward, actual or potential problems can be identified and care planned accordingly. It must be noted, however, that if a patient has been pre-assessed this does not negate the need for a comprehensive and ongoing assessment once the patient is admitted to a ward or day unit.

It can be seen from the diagram that patient assessment is not a single event. The information gathering process does not cease there. Patient assessment and planning of patient care is a dynamic process. Each stage should be negotiated with the patient and outcomes evaluated against certain goals and measures. The information gained during evaluation restarts the whole cycle.

Planning patient care

As previously, a great deal of information may be gained during the phase of patient assessment. However, in order to plan appropriate care some method of identifying actual or potential problems is required. Since the late 1960s many nursing theorists have identified various views on nursing and their philosophies of care. Emerging from this was the concept of models of nursing. These provide a framework to process the information available, and relate the care required to the needs of the patient.

Many models of nursing are in existence today, however for the purpose of this chapter Roper's model of nursing will be used in order to identify problems and plan patient care. Although often viewed as simplistic, *The Activities of Daily Living* is still commonly used both within hospital and educational settings. This chapter does not propose to examine the model in detail but to utilise it to demonstrate some of the issues encountered whilst caring for the patient undergoing oral and maxillofacial surgery.

Pre- and post-operative nursing issues

Maintaining a safe environment

Preparation of the bedside area

In order to provide the best possible standard of care it is important to ensure that the area in which the patient will be nursed is organised appropriately. Oxygen and suction equipment should be properly maintained. It may be useful to have a selection of suction heads and suction catheters near to hand, for example Yankeur and Sims suckers. Furthermore, it is often useful to have a small tray at the patient's bedside with some gloves, gauze and swabs for routine cases, should they be required. These trays can be adapted according to the procedure that the patient will undergo, for example mouth wash and mouth care equipment for those experiencing major oral surgery.

It is important to recognise that in preparing the area for post-operative care, further anxieties may be provoked in the patient. However this preparation provides the nursing staff with an opportunity to explore pre-operative anxieties, allay fears and give explanations about what to expect post-operatively. There are many studies which reinforce this principle of information giving to reduce anxieties, thus providing a less eventful post-operative recovery period.

Preparation for surgery

In addition to the provision of appropriate information for the patient, the nurse, as for any surgical patient, should ensure that the pre-operative check list is completed accurately. To prevent delays and problems in theatre, the nurse must ascertain that the appropriate and recent test results, X-rays and operation consent have been obtained and are available to the surgical team.

If one examines the activity of 'maintaining a safe environment' in relation to post-operative care other issues are raised.

General observations

During the assessment phase of patient care a baseline set of vital signs observations should be made, against which post-operative observations can be monitored. It is essential to ensure that the patient remains haemodynamically stable, thus assessment of the patient's pulse, blood pressure and temperature should be made frequently in the early post-operative phase of care. However, the need for continual observation must be assessed according to the nature and extent of the operation performed.

In addition to vital signs monitoring, the nurse should also observe the patient for swelling. To prevent excessive swelling and assist in the natural dispersion of oedema it is advisable to nurse the patient in an upright position, as soon as their haemodynamic condition allows. This will also help prevent any further complications such as excessive discomfort or, in extreme cases, airway obstruction from occurring.

Pain control

Pain control is also a priority for any post-operative patient. For routine operations, simple analgesics are usually sufficient. However, it must be remembered that each person has a different perception of pain, hence individualised assessment is required. Patients undergoing more major operations may benefit from patient controlled analgesic systems in the immediate post-operative phase of care, whilst those experiencing pain from tumours may benefit from opioid analgesics such as modified morphine preparations.

Prevention of infection

Prevention of infection is another basic aim of post-operative care. The conditions in the mouth provide an ideal environment for bacteria to multiply and any wound is susceptible. The importance of good oral care pre- and post- operatively cannot be overlooked. Regular mouthwashes and cleaning of teeth should be encouraged, to reduce the risk of infection. Although relatively uncommon in current practice, particular attention should be paid to the patient with their jaws wired together. In this instance the patient should be encouraged to clean their teeth with a soft toothbrush. A 50 ml syringe is often useful for the patient to rinse out their inner mouth. Removal of debris is aided by syringing the mouthwash behind the wired teeth, and asking the patient to lean forward, allowing the fluid to drain. Many external wounds of the head and neck area require only simple gauze dressings until the initial oozing has ceased, after which they can be left uncovered.

Wound drainage and bleeding

Efficient drainage of wounds in the head and neck area is most important as inefficient drainage may result in the following complications due to haematoma formation:

- Airway obstruction
- Loss of flaps
- Wound dehiscence or infection

Drainage must be observed and recorded, and action taken if excessive or sudden drainage or swelling occurs. If such a situation does arise then sutures or staples can be removed to assist is the dispersion of the hae-matoma.

As with any surgical operation, the patient is at risk of bleeding post-operatively. Excessive oozing or bleeding must be reported and stemmed as soon as possible. Bleeding from intra-oral wounds is usually controlled by pressure exerted by an appropriately placed gauze swab, and should cease after several minutes. However if the bleeding continues further investigation may be required.

It is often advisable to ask patients returning from theatre after surgery with mouth packs in position to remove them themselves once they are fully alert and the pack becomes uncomfortable or irritating to them.

Eating and drinking

Eating and drinking is another 'activity of daily living' which has parti-cular relevance in the care of patients undergoing oral and maxillofacial surgery.

Dietary requirements

Once the patient has returned from surgery and is both stable and com-fortable, they should be encouraged to begin taking as normal a diet as possible. Often it is advisable to provide analgesics prior to eating, especially for those having undergone intra-oral operations. Good mouth care should be encouraged after food intake. In some instances it will be necessary to provide a soft or liquidised diet, for example for patients post-osteotomy or following fracture treatment. Enteral feeding (naso-gastric tube or gastrostomy) may be required for patients undergoing major ablative and reconstructive procedures. Input from the dietetic department is essential for these cases.

Fluid balance

Accurate maintenance of fluid balance charts is essential for patients on intravenous fluids. Similarly, patients being fed enterally must also have their intake and output recorded accurately. This ensures that the patient is receiving adequate hydration without being fluid overloaded and, in the case of enteral feeding, that adequate nutrition is being provided.

Communicating

Patients in the initial post operative phase of care often experience diffi-culty in communicating for a number of reasons. Local anaesthetics may inhibit oral competence, thus the patient may experience drooling of saliva. In most cases this is a temporary impairment and will resolve spontaneously. However for patients undergoing major ablative and reconstructive surgery speech therapy may be required to assist them to gain control post-operatively.

Pain may also inhibit communication, and nursing staff should ensure adequate pain relief is available and allow patients time to communicate their needs effectively.

Working and playing

The main aim of care for the patient is for them to resume their normal life as quickly as possible, and careful and appropriate discharge planning should be made.

Discharge planning

If possible the patient's discharge should be discussed at the time of pre-admission assessment. Many routine cases are treated as day patients, and it is important to ensure that the appropriate information is conveyed to and understood by the patient and accompanying person. Verbal information backed up with written documentation is advisable. Out-patient appointments and discharge medication should also be explained to the patient. Where possible it is best to give discharge information well before the patient leaves the ward area, allowing for any questions to be answered.

For those patients undergoing major surgery, liaison with other members of the multidisciplinary team, for example the head and neck Macmillan nurse, may also be required to facilitate the smooth transition from hospital to home or hospice care. Other support groups, such as BACUP and Changing Faces, may also be useful in providing information and support for the patient and their family.

Summary

- Patient assessment at pre-admission clinics must be supported by further assessment of physical and psychological needs in order to provide appropriate patient care.
- Patient assessment, planning, implementing and evaluating care form an ongoing process which is dynamic in nature.
- The use of a nursing model helps in the structuring of care planning.
- General principles of care remain the same for many operations.
- Referral to other members of the multidisciplinary team may be required in order to provide the most appropriate care for the individual.

Examples of care plans

SURGICAL REMOVAL OF IMPACTED WISDOM TEETH CARE PLAN

Name of patient . . . . HOSPITAL TRUST

Hospital Number . . . .

Date	Problem	Goal	Interventions	Rationale	Date resolved	Signature of nurse
	Patient at pre-assessment or on admission	To reduce anxiety	Explain to the patient prior to the operation all procedures and rationale. Allow time for questions and answer as appropriate	To ensure understanding and provide information		
	Patient has undergone removal of impacted wisdom teeth	To reduce swelling and prevent bleeding	Observe vital signs until stable . . . . hourly	To observe change and ensure stability		
			Encourage the patient to be nursed sitting up as soon as possible	Reduces oozing and swelling		
			Ensure dental pack is *in situ*. Remove when bleeding or oozing has ceased. Removed at . . . . If bleeding continues, replace pack and apply pressure to the bleeding point	Pressure helps to prevent bleeding		
		To promote comfort	Administer analgesics as prescribed			
			Place ice packs			
		To prevent infection	Encourage good oral hygiene	Ensures the wound/socket is kept clean, reducing the risk of infection and encouraging rapid healing		
			Commence hot salty mouth washes 24 hours post-operatively			

Fig. 3.1   Care plan for removal of impacted wisdom teeth.

. . . . **HOSPITAL TRUST**

NECK DISSECTION CARE PLAN

Name of patient . . . .   **Hospital Number** . . . .

Date	Problem	Goal	Interventions	Rationale	Date resolved	Signature of nurse
	Patient admitted for major surgery	To reduce anxiety	Explain to the patient all procedures and rationale prior to the operation. Allow time for questions	To ensure understanding and provide information		
	Patient has undergone neck dissection	To promote healing and comfort	Observe vital signs hourly until stable and 4 hourly thereafter	To observe change and ensure stability		
			Observe wound drainage 6–12 hourly and chart as appropriate	To prevent formation of haematoma		
			Liaise with medical staff on drain removal	Drains usually removed when drainage is <20 ml/24 hours		
			Nurse patient sitting up as soon as possible	To allow gravity to reduce oedema and protect airway		
			Observe suture line and cleanse as required	Prevention of infection		
			Remove sutures on			

Fig. 3.2(a)   Care plan for neck dissection.

.... **HOSPITAL TRUST**

NECK DISSECTION CARE PLAN

Name of patient ....   Hospital Number ....

Date	Problem	Goal	Interventions	Rationale	Date resolved	Signature of nurse
	Patient may be experiencing pain	To alleviate pain and promote comfort	Assess the level, intensity and site of the pain experienced	To promote comfort		
			Administer appropriate analgesics as indicated and prescribed			
			Assist patient into a comfortable position using appropriate lifting and handling techniques			
	Potential problem due to decreased mobility and duration of operation	To prevent complications and promote independence	Monitor respiration rate, especially if the patient is using a PCA pump	To prevent narcotic induced respiratory depression		
			Encourage the patient to practise deep breathing and coughing exercises. Liaise with the physiotherapist	To prevent chest infection		
			Encourage the patient to participate in active leg exercises	To prevent formation of deep vein thrombosis		
			Ensure that the patient is wearing anti-embolism stockings			
			Observe pressure areas and ensure appropriate pressure relieving device is in place	To prevent pressure sores		

Fig. 3.2(b)   Care plan for neck dissection.

MAJOR FLAP CARE PLAN

Name of patient . . . .   **HOSPITAL TRUST**

Hospital Number . . . .

Date	Problem	Goal	Interventions	Rationale	Date resolved	Signature of nurse
	Patient admitted for major surgery	To reduce anxiety	Explain to the patient all procedures and rationale prior to the operation. Allow time for questions	To ensure understanding and provide information		
	Patient has undergone major flap surgery. Potential problem of the flap not surviving	To maintain viability of the flap, prevent complications and promote comfort	Observe vital signs hourly, decrease to 4 hourly when observations are stable	To observe change and ensure stability		
			Nurse patient in warm environment. Maintain body temperature >37°C	Encourage vasodilatation and blood flow		
			Observe flap hourly for colour, warmth, sensation and capillary return, only decreasing observations when the flap becomes stable	Ensure flap survival		
			Observe hydration status. If patient is catheterised, observe the urine output hourly. Maintain an accurate fluid input and output chart. Administer IV fluids and antibiotics as prescribed	Ideally the patient should be slightly haemodiluted		
			Ensure that dressings around the flap are kept clean and dry			

Fig. 3.3(a)   Care plan for major flap surgery.

MAJOR FLAP CARE PLAN

Name of patient . . . . HOSPITAL TRUST

Hospital Number . . . .

Date	Problem	Goal	Interventions	Rationale	Date resolved	Signature of nurse
	Patient may be experiencing pain	To alleviate pain and promote comfort	Assess the level, intensity and site of the pain experienced	To promote comfort		
			Administer appropriate analgesics as indicated and prescribed			
			Assist patient into a comfortable position using appropriate lifting and handling techniques			
	Potential problem due to decreased mobility and duration of operation	To prevent complications and promote independence	Monitor respiration rate, especially if the patient is using a PCA pump	To prevent narcotic induced respiratory depression		
			Encourage the patient to practise deep breathing and coughing exercises. Liaise with the physiotherapist	To prevent chest infection		
			Encourage the patient to participate in active leg exercises	To prevent formation of deep vein thrombosis		
			Ensure that the patient is wearing anti-embolism stockings			
			Observe pressure areas and ensure appropriate pressure relieving device is in place	To prevent pressure sores		

Fig. 3.3(b)   Care plan for major flap surgery.

DAY PATIENT RECORD

CHILDREN'S UNIT

Fig. 3.4 Care plan for children for day surgery.

Date of pre-clerking:	Date of admission:
Pre-admission programme attended YES/NO	Time of admission:
Hospital label (Name/Address/Hosp No/DoB) NHS No: Telephone No: Consultant	Diagnosis/Operation Child's understanding of operation Parent's understanding of operation
Age Religion HV School	GP Label
NoK/Relationship Address	Immunisations DPT Polio HIB MMR Pre-school booster BCG Rubella Other
2nd Contact Telephone	Contact with infectious diseases in the past month:
Past Medical History/Admissions Operations	Medications Allergies
CPR REGISTER YES/NO	

DAY CASE ASSESSMENT AND CARE PLAN

NAME DOB	HOSPITAL NUMBER WARD
CHILD'S USUAL NAME / /	
COMMUNICATION	PRE-OPERATIVE CARE NEGOTIATED WITH
	. . . .

LANGUAGE   SPEECH
                HEARING
                SIGHT
	RELATION TO CHILD/TEENAGER

INTERPRETER NEEDED YES/NO	PARENTAL CONSENT OBTAINED FOR NURSING DOCUMENTATION TO BE HELD AT BEDSIDE
	YES [ ] NO [ ]
BREATHING	NURSE TAKING HISTORY
BREATHING PROBLEMS E.G. ASTHMA	DESIGNATION
HISTORY OF GENERAL ANAESTHETIC YES/NO	PRIMARY NURSE
ANY PROBLEMS YES/NO	SIGNATURE
TEMPERATURE	
HAVE YOU ANY PARACETAMOL AT HOME YES/NO	

PERSONAL CLEANSING	**PLAY PREPARATION**
ANY SKIN PROBLEMS E.G. ECZEMA YES/NO	PREPARED BY:
LEISURE AND PLAYING	Preparation aids used:
FAVOURITE TOY/COMFORTER	Doll [ ] Book [ ] Play [ ] Story [ ] Puppets [ ] Photographs [ ]
SAFE ENVIRONMENT	Play People [ ] Explanation [ ]
SLEEPS IN BED/COT	Other [ ]
MOBILISING	Visit to Dept YES [ ] NO [ ]
ANY MOBILITY PROBLEMS? YES/NO	Ward facilities explained to parents YES [ ] NO [ ]
EATING Time	COMMENTS
NIL BY MOUTH SINCE Food Clear Fluids	Specific fears/anxieties recorded and made known to relevant carers?
. . . . . . will ensure . . . . . is NBM as instructed	YES [ ] NO [ ]
PERSONAL WORRIES	Please state:
ANY PARTICULAR FEARS OR WORRIES YES/NO	

DAY CASE CARE PLAN FOR . . . . DATE: . . . .

NURSING GOAL: To provide safe, planned care and discharge home in 10 hrs.

PROBLEM/NEED	NURSING ACTION	TIME	EVALUATION	SIG
1. . . . . and family are unfamiliar with ward environment and perioperative procedures.	Orientate family to ward. Ensure all perioperative procedures are explained and understood by parents/child. Ask parents if they wish to accompany to and from theatre. Record baseline TPR/weight/BP.			
2. Child will benefit from parental involvement in care.	Negotiate share care with parents.			
3. . . . . needs to be safely prepared for theatre.	Complete theatre check list. Inform Dr/Anaesthetist of any problems.			
4. . . . . needs safe transfer from theatre to ward.	Ensure there is working O_2 and suction for transfer and at bedside for return. Ensure cot sides up for safe transfer.			

NAME:			DATE:	
RETURNED FROM THEATRE AT . . . . *HOURS*				
PROBLEM NEED	*NURSING ACTION*	*TIME*	*EVALUATION*	*SIG*
5. Due to surgery . . . . is at risk of breathing difficulties, haemorrhage and infection.	As condition warrants: – record pulse and respirations $\frac{1}{2}$ hrly until fully awake. – report if outside normal limits (limits . . . .) – record temp, ensure temperature within normal limits (36.0–37.5°C axilla) before discharge. – record BP if appropriate – observe wound site . . . . for any bleeding/discharge. – wound care/dressing if required.			
6. . . . . is at risk of dehydration, nausea/vomiting following anaesthetic/surgery.	Give nil orally until fully awake. Nursing staff to supervise parents offering sips of clear fluids, increasing to free fluids/diet once tolerated. Record any vomiting. Ensure child has passed urine before discharge.			
7. . . . . may have pain following surgery.	After discussion with . . . . use . . . . pain chart to assess degree of pain and monitor effectiveness of analgesia.			
8. Parents/carers need to understand care required on discharge home.	Ensure . . . . is seen by doctor post-operatively and discharge plan is completed.			

COMMUNICATION SHEET

Date		Signature & Designation

POST-OPERATIVE TELEPHONE QUESTIONNAIRE

Tick appropriate answer: No answer   [   ]   Line engaged   [   ]   Re-tried at . . . .

Message left on answerphone   [   ]

Mark appropriate answer. Comment if necessary.

How is the child today: normal self/quiet/sleepy/other		
Are they eating/drinking as normal	YES	NO
Have they been sick since discharge	YES	NO
If yes, how many times: once/twice/three times/more than three times		
Does the wound appear alright, e.g. bleeding/discharge/redness	YES	NO
Do you think they are in any pain	YES	NO
Are you giving them any medicine for the pain	YES	NO
If yes, what medicine and how often		
Is the medicine relieving the pain	YES	NO
Is there anything else you are worried about	YES	NO
If yes, state what		
If we had not telephoned, would you have contacted anyone else	YES	NO
If yes, state who		
Advice given		
Refer to PCNs		
Date: Name: Signature:		

DISCHARGE PLAN

FULL NAME . . . .   CONSULTANT . . . .

HOSPITAL No . . . .   PRIMARY NURSE . . . .

DoB   /   /19   DISCHARGE DATE   /   /19

ADMISSION DATE   /   /19   DESTINATION . . . .

WARD . . . .

Details you need to know	Actions taken	Date & Signature
Medication: 1. Self/parent medication discharge form complete 2. Medicines to take home are:	YES / NO	
Out-patient appointment: (additional investigations, physio, dietitian, X-ray)	Time: Date: Place:	
Community referral: Community Paediatric Nurse or Asthma Nurse	YES / NO	
GP/GP Nurse	YES / NO	
Do you require transport?	YES / NO	
GP Information: Discharge letter Surgery informed	YES / NO YES / NO	
Health Visitor: Referral form completed/contracted Parent held record book/continuation sheet completed	YES / NO YES / NO	
School Nurse: Form completed/Contacted	YES / NO	
Social Services Referral:	YES / NO	
Information/teaching received prior to . . . . discharge (include any information sheets/policies given)		
Cannula removed:	YES / NO	
What to do in the event of an emergency:		

Please contact the Ward if you have any problems or concerns. Telephone . . . .

I fully understand and agree with the information above.

Teenager/Parent's signature . . . .

Nurse's signature . . . . Date . . . .

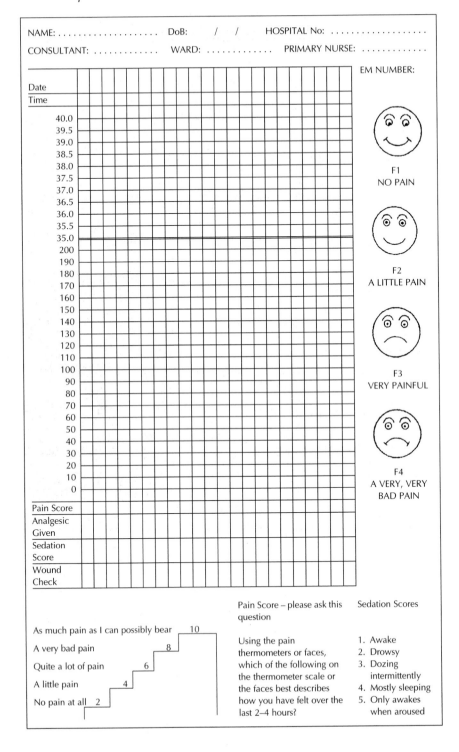

NAME: . . . .   DoB: /   /   HOSPITAL No: . . . .

CONSULTANT: . . . .   WARD: . . . .   PRIMARY NURSE: . . . .

EM NUMBER:

Date

Time

40.0
39.5
39.0
38.5
38.0
37.5
37.0
36.5
36.0
35.5
35.0
200
190
180
170
160
150
140
130
120
110
100
90
80
70
60
50
40
30
20
10
0

Pain Score

Analgesic Given

Sedation Score

Wound Check

F1
NO PAIN

F2
A LITTLE PAIN

F3
VERY PAINFUL

F4
A VERY, VERY
BAD PAIN

As much pain as I can possibly bear   10

A very bad pain   8

Quite a lot of pain   6

A little pain   4

No pain at all   2

Pain Score – please ask this question

Using the pain thermometers or faces, which of the following on the thermometer scale or the faces best describes how you have felt over the last 2–4 hours?

Sedation Scores

1. Awake
2. Drowsy
3. Dozing intermittently
4. Mostly sleeping
5. Only awakes when aroused

4

Operating Theatre

M. Slater

This chapter covers the role of the nurse working in the oral and maxillofacial surgery operating theatre. It assumes familiarity with the general duties and responsibilities of any operating theatre nurse, and concentrates on aspects specific to the specialty.

Patient check-in and identification

- Routine admission procedures will have taken place, but on arrival in the theatre unit the patient's identification must be cross-checked with the notes and the theatre list.
- The patient is asked their name (parent/guardian in the case of a child) and this must correspond with the rest of the cross-checking.
- The patient's wrist band must also be checked against name, date of birth, hospital number, etc.
- Allergies must be noted and reported to both anaesthetist and surgeon.
- Jewellery should have been removed or secured with tape.
- Dentures and other prostheses should be removed prior to arrival in theatre. Hearing aids are often best left in place until the patient is anaesthetised and then handed to recovery staff with the patient's identification attached, to be reinserted when the patient is waking up.
- Nil by mouth status needs to be checked as well as the last time food and drink were taken.
- The operation consent form must have been completed and signed by the clinician and patient (or parent/guardian) prior to administration of premedication or anaesthetic.
- Any final queries from the patient or parent/guardian should be made before the commencement of the anaesthetic.

Preparation and positioning of patient

- Due to the nature of oral and maxillofacial surgery (OMFS), in most cases throat packs will be inserted by the anaesthetist after intubation and prior to the start of surgery. The anaesthetist records this in the notes and ensures removal at the end of the procedure. For some procedures, however, a laryngeal mask is suitable. Eyes are routinely protected with well secured eye pads. The endotracheal tube will need to be very well secured as access is difficult once the patient has been draped.
- With the anaesthetist's agreement the patient should be transferred to the operating table in a safe manner, with particular care taken not to disrupt anaesthetic tubes, lines, etc.
- The anaesthetic machine needs to be positioned at the opposite end to the patient's head, about hip/thigh level is usually ideal for both surgeon and anaesthetist, but this does necessitate extra long anaesthetic tubing.
- With the anaesthetist's permission, the patient's head is stabilised on a suitable head rest and the circulating nurse/ODA/technician attaches a diathermy plate (if needed).

- If surgery on the neck is to be performed a shoulder bar may also be needed to extend the patient's neck to allow easier access for the surgeon. The head is rotated away from the side of operation. Special care must be taken with elderly or arthritic patients to ensure the head and neck are not overextended or unstable. This group may also require extra padding to prevent excessive pressure on prominent bony areas.
- Arms should be placed by the patient's side and held in place with padded arm retainers.
- Anti-embolic protection must be used on the patient's legs to prevent stasis of blood, particularly in longer cases.
- Other routine care and protection of the patient should be taken as for all surgery.

Operating site

Preparation

Depending on the site of surgery and sex of the patient, it may be necessary to shave an appropriate area, and loose hair must then be cleared away to ensure it does not contaminate the operation site. The skin is prepared according to the surgeon's preference. Aqueous solutions are recommended for skin preparation.

Draping

Two suitable sized drapes are placed under the patient's head. The appropriate area for surgery is prepared according to the surgeon's preference, and the upper drape wrapped around the head leaving the surgical field exposed. Absorbent disposable sterile material such as cotton wool or gamgee can be placed beside the neck on one or both sides to help absorb any blood or fluid should the case warrant it. The patient's body and neck are then covered with a large drape for intra-oral surgery. Two side drapes can be used to expose more of the surgical field for extra-oral surgery, alternatively a large U-drape can be used to cover body and sides in one.

Set-up

The scrub nurse should then connect suction apparatus (and diathermy if required) and ensure it is switched on ready for the start of surgery. The surgeon indicates where the lights need to be positioned. The final adjustment of the lighting is best done by the surgeon or assistant using sterile light handles.

Instrument technique

It is the scrub nurse's responsibility to maintain swab, needle and instrument counts during the operation and to ensure that all instruments are kept clean and well organised. Dirty instruments are not only difficult to use, but also risk contaminating the operation site. For major surgery it may be useful to place a sterile magnetic mat on the patient's chest on top of the drapes to prevent instruments from slipping. It also reduces the risk of injury to the patient should the surgeon inadvertently put a sharp instrument down before the scrub nurse can retrieve it.

During closure a final swab, needle and instrument count is made.

Positions for scrub nurse and trolley

Surgery with one surgeon

The scrub nurse, who may also be acting as assistant, should stand opposite the surgeon with the instrument trolley across the head of the table, allowing them both access to the trolley (Fig. 4.1).

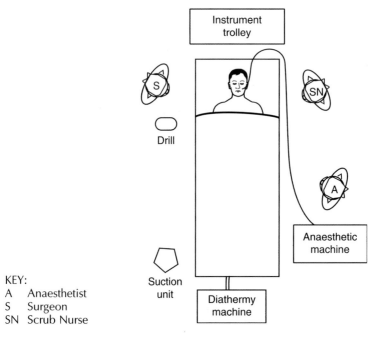

KEY:
A   Anaesthetist
S   Surgeon
SN   Scrub Nurse

Fig. 4.1   Positions for surgery with one surgeon.

Surgery with surgeon and assistant

There are two positions depending on the surgery to be performed:

(1) Scrub nurse at the head of the patient facing the patient's feet, with the instrument trolley at her side (Fig. 4.2).
(2) If the surgeon or assistant is standing at the patient's head the scrub nurse can stand on the free side with the instrument trolley in front of her (Fig. 4.3).

Both these positions allow for a second instrument trolley to be placed at right angles to the first, keeping the first trolley as the working trolley and maintaining a sterile field.

Surgery with surgeon and more than one assistant

The best position for the scrub nurse is to stand at about the patient's hip level on the opposite side to the anaesthetic machine with her working

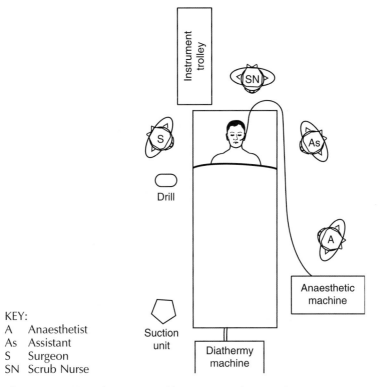

KEY:
A   Anaesthetist
As   Assistant
S   Surgeon
SN   Scrub Nurse

Fig. 4.2 Positions for surgery with surgeon and one assistant.

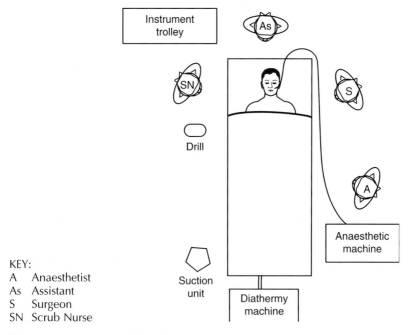

Fig. 4.3 Alternative positions for surgery with surgeon and one assistant.

trolley in front and other trolleys to the side. This allows the surgeon and assistants to move around without disrupting the scrub nurse (Fig. 4.4).

Procedure at conclusion of surgery

At the conclusion of surgery it is essential that the oral cavity is cleared by suction and carefully checked for any remaining debris. Following this the throat pack is removed and the oro-pharynx inspected and cleared if necessary. The anaesthetist may also wish to check the pharynx using a laryngoscope.

It is the scrub nurse's responsibility to ensure that a verbal handover of the patient to the recovery nurse takes place, prior to the completion of relevant theatre documentation. Trolleys and instruments are then cleared away and the operating theatre reset.

Recovery room practice

General

This will not be described in detail, but routine observations are as follows:

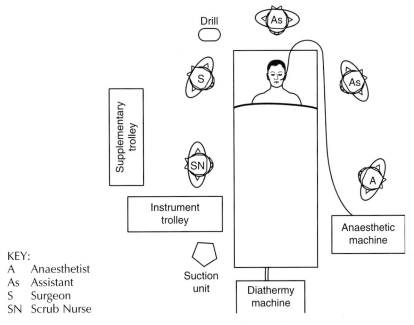

Fig. 4.4   Positions for surgery with surgeon and more than one assistant.

- Airway maintenance and administration of oxygen
- Oxygen saturation monitoring
- Pulse and blood pressure
- Respiratory rate
- Conscious level and observation of reflexes
- Wound site and drains

Specific to OMFS

- Airway management in recovery is always important, but particular care is necessary with a patient who has undergone surgery involving any part of the airway.
- Oro-pharyngeal airways are frequently used and their patency must be ensured at all times, with jaw support when necessary. Naso-pharyngeal airways may be placed by the anaesthetist as a useful alternative following surgery for fractures of the jaws, osteotomies and any surgery where the jaws may be fixed together.
- Many patients will have been placed in a lateral position initially.
- Oral packs are usually placed following routine oral surgery to reduce oozing and prevent blood from being swallowed. Their presence must be recorded and they normally remain in place until the patient returns to the ward.

- Efficient aspiration equipment is essential and must be used when removal of secretions, blood or vomit is necessary.
- Observations for excessive swallowing should be made as this could indicate bleeding which can sometimes be difficult to diagnose in the early stages after certain types of surgery where there are no external wounds.
- Post-operatively these patients should be positioned head up when routine observations are stable, and this position maintained on the ward. This is not only more comfortable for the patient, but also reduces post-operative swelling and improves the patient's breathing.
- If the jaws have been fixed together, wire cutters must be immediately available for release of the fixation if airway obstruction occurs.
- Some patients will need to be transferred directly from the operating theatre to an intensive care or high dependency unit.

Operation, use and maintenance of equipment

Surgical instruments

These will be cleaned, lubricated, repacked and autoclaved after use according to local practice.

Care of drills and saws

- These pieces of equipment should always be maintained, cleaned and oiled according to manufacturers' instructions. Not only will this ensure that equipment lasts longer, but also that any problems such as stiff or sticking joints, damaged hoses, etc., are detected and corrected or repaired at an early stage. When training staff in the setting up, use and maintenance of new or existing equipment it is essential to explain why all the care and steps are taken, as far greater learning and acceptance of procedures are achieved than if the 'we always do it this way' method is used.
- If air driven instruments are used the air supply should be positioned conveniently for surgery. The hoses should be checked to ensure they are compatible with the air pipelines, if available, or the cylinders if these are used. Spare air cylinders should be available for quick changeover should the first run out.
- The power cables of electrically driven instruments must be of a suitable length to facilitate easy use and avoid causing a hazard with trailing cables.

Irrigation

If needed this should be set up in advance to ensure that the procedure is not delayed. When used it will be the circulating nurse's duty to ensure it does not run dry and to replenish the fluid as and when required, informing the scrub nurse if switching off is necessary.

Suction

The importance of efficient suction throughout these procedures cannot be overemphasised. It must be connected immediately after draping the patient and should not be disconnected until the patient leaves the operating theatre.

It is essential to ensure that suction tubing is long enough to be used at the operating site and to be connected to its source by the patient's feet – 3 m is the ideal length.

Suction bottles or liners may need to be replaced during an operation, and it is the runner's duty to ensure that a replacement is available, and to inform the scrub nurse and surgeon that there will be a temporary loss of suction when the changeover is taking place. The anaesthetist will require both the scrub nurse and runner to keep a careful note of the irrigation used so that blood loss can be calculated.

If a disposable pharyngeal suction end is supplied to the scrub nurse at the start of the procedure, this can be connected to the suction tubing at the end of surgery for the anaesthetist to use during extubation, thus utilising existing equipment and saving the cost of a length of suction tubing, and cleaning or replacing a suction liner.

Efficient suction is essential for safe, expeditious surgery. The removal of blood, debris and irrigation fluid from the operative field improves operator vision and promotes uncomplicated healing.

Instrumentation

The following sets show the instruments that are required for a variety of surgery included in this book, although each hospital and surgeon will have their own preferences. Sponge holders, towel clips, etc., have been omitted so as not to clutter the photographs. General tissue sets have not been included as these tend to be standard to most surgery in most hospitals (Figs 4.5 to 4.14).

Microsurgical instruments

Instruments for microsurgery are expensive, delicate and must be in immaculate condition. Each instrument should have a protective tip cover. After use, each should be cleaned with a warm detergent solution, thoroughly dried, the protective cap placed over the tip and the complete set stored in a ventilated box to avoid corrosion. Regular demagnetisation is required to prevent inadvertent 'picking up' of microneedles and

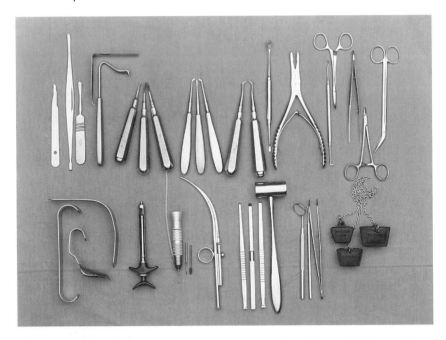

Fig. 4.5   Surgical tray No 1: this is comprehensive and can be modified according to preference and the procedure to be undertaken. *Top row* (left to right): scalpel (No 15 blade), periosteal elevator (Howarth), periosteal elevator (Fickling), Austin retractor, rake retractor, Coupland chisels, Warwick James elevators, Cryers elevators, bone file, bone nibblers, Mitchells trimmer, mosquito forceps, dissecting forceps, scissors and needle holder. *Bottom row* (left to right): cheek retractor, upper third molar retractor, tongue retractor, local anaesthetic syringe, straight handpiece and burs, self-clearing sucker, chisels, osteotome and mallet, mirror, probe and tweezers, mouth props.

secondary magnetisation of clamps, etc. during surgery. A typical set of microsurgery instruments is listed below.

JF.3 Jeweller's forceps × 2
JF.5 Jeweller's forceps × 2
D5AZ Vessel dilator × 1
104 Suture tying forceps STR. 6″ × 1
167 Microscissors STR. 6″ × 1
068 Microscissors CVD. 6″ × 1
035 Microneedleholder CVD. 6″ × 1
CAF.4 Clamp applying forceps × 1

C.B.1 Clamp box × 1
Acland microclamps 2A × 2
Acland microclamps 2V × 4
Acland microclamps 3A x 2
Acland microclamps 3V × 2
Acland microclamps HD-S × 2
Acland microclamps RD-S × 2
E4026/4 Sterilising container × 1

Most microsurgeons use 8/0 nylon sutures.

Instruments for temporomandibular joint arthroscopy and surgery

See Chapter 10.

Summary

The theatre nurse's importance in the delivery of a high quality specialty service cannot be overemphasised. As far as possible smooth running should be achieved by standardising procedures, while maintaining sufficient flexibility to accommodate inevitable variations in clinical practice. Patient safety must take priority at all times.

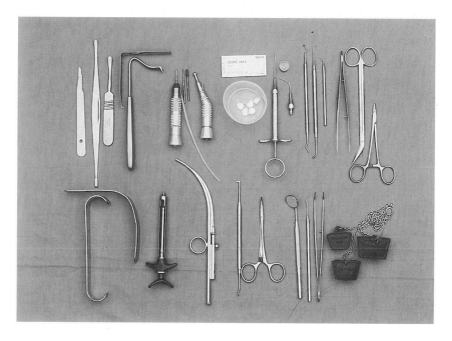

Fig. 4.6 Surgical tray No 2: for periapical surgery. *Top row* (left to right): scalpel (No 15 blade), periosteal elevator (Howarth), periosteal elevator (Fickling), Austin retractor, rake retractor, straight handpiece with burs, retrograde handpiece, bone wax and cotton wool pledgelets, amalgam carrier and amalgam holder, excavator and amalgam pluggers, dissecting forceps, scissors and needle holders. *Bottom row* (left to right): cheek retractor, tongue retractor, local anaesthetic syringe, self-clearing sucker, Mitchell's trimmer, mosquito forceps, mirror, probe, college tweezers, mouth props.

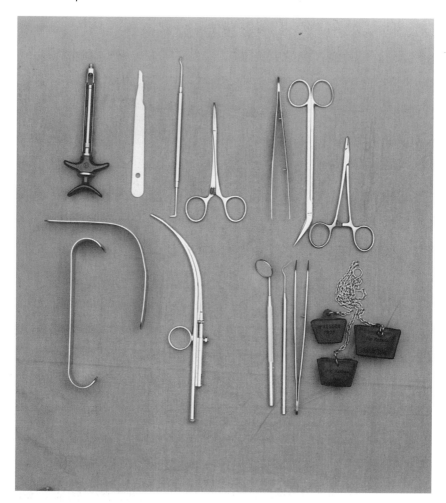

Fig. 4.7   Surgical tray No 3: soft tissue and biopsy. *Top row* (left to right): local anaesthetic syringe, scalpel (No 15 blade), Mitchells trimmer, mosquito forceps, dissecting forceps, scissors and needle holder. *Bottom row* (left to right): cheek retractor, tongue retractor, self-clearing sucker, mirror, probe and tweezers, mouth props.

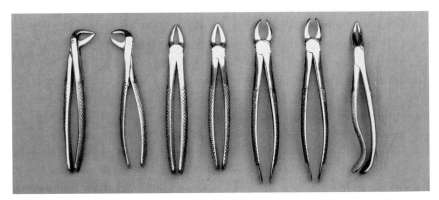

Fig. 4.8 Extraction forceps (left to right): lower root forceps, lower crown forceps, upper straight forceps, upper root forceps, upper molar forceps (right), upper molar forceps (left), bayonet forceps.

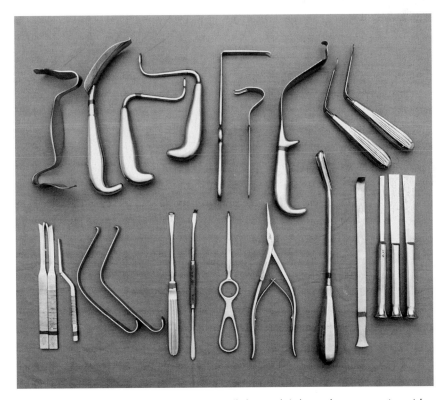

Fig. 4.9 Osteotomy instruments. *Top row* (left to right): buccal retractor, sigmoid notch retractor, maxillary mobilisers, forked retractor, chin retractor, ramus retractor, channel retractor. *Bottom row* (left to right): nasal chisels, channel retractors (Obwegeser), periosteal strippers, bone hook, bone separating forceps, long channel retractor, pterygoid chisel, osteotomes.

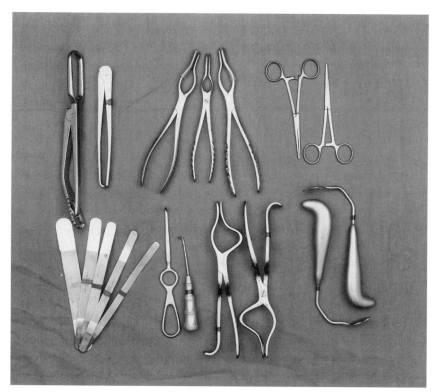

Fig. 4.10   Fracture set. *Top row* (left to right): Rowe zygomatic elevator, Kilner zygomatic elevator, nasal reduction forceps, Kocher forceps. *Bottom row* (left to right): malleable strip retractors, bone hooks, maxillary disimpaction forceps, orbital floor retractors.

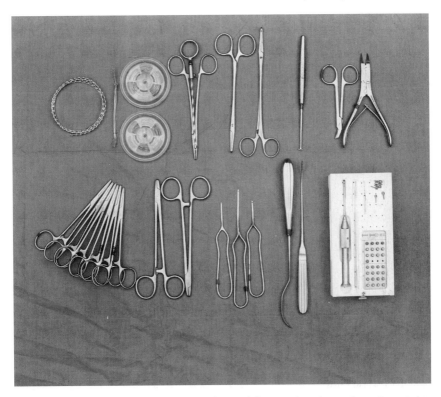

Fig. 4.11   Wiring set. *Top row* (left to right): arch bar, eyelet wires, wire, wire twisting forceps, wire passing forceps, boat hook for elastics, wire cutters. *Bottom row* (left to right): wire holding forceps, wire tightening forceps, bone awls, soft tissue awls, bone pin system for intermaxillary fixation.

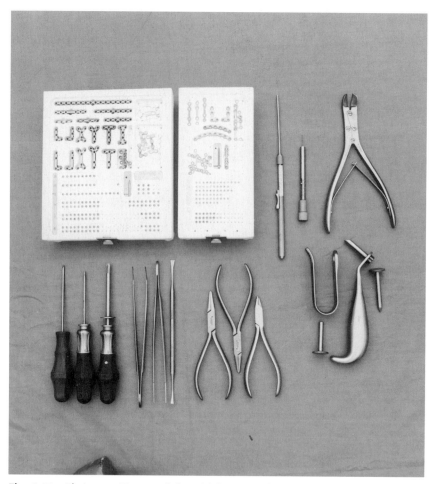

Fig;. 4.12   Plating set. *Top row* (left to right): mini and micro plates and screws, depth gauges (long and short), plate cutters. *Bottom row* (left to right): screwdrivers, plate holding forceps, plate holding fork, plate bending pliers, percutaneous instruments.

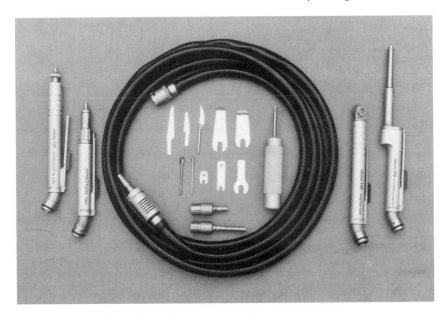

Fig. 4.13 Air powered drill/saw system.

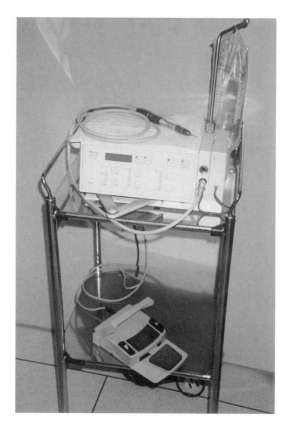

Fig. 4.14   Surgical drill.

5

Dentoalveolar Surgery

T.J. Storrs and C. Yates

This chapter describes the most commonly performed procedures in dentoalveolar surgery. Procedures generally are described in terms of indications and aims, the procedure itself, aftercare and complications.

Dentoalveolar procedures

Dentoalveolar surgery is the surgery of the tooth bearing portions of the jaws. The alveolus is the part of the jaw which normally contains and supports the roots of the teeth (*see* Fig. C in the Introduction). Gradual atrophy of the alveolus takes place following loss of teeth.

Adjacent structures which may be involved in any disease process affecting the alveolus, or in surgery to the alveolus, are:

■ The soft tissues of the mouth and face and associated nerves and blood vessels.
■ In the mandible: the neurovascular canal running beneath the roots of the premolar and molar teeth.
■ In the maxilla: the nasal and antral cavities.

With the exception of dental extractions the most commonly performed dentoalveolar procedure is the removal of impacted third molars (wisdom teeth). The requirement for this procedure to be performed in large numbers of young adults (over a quarter of a million cases yearly in England and Wales) makes it highly significant in socio-economic terms.

The bulk of dentoalveolar surgery is carried out on an out-patient basis under local anaesthetic (with sedation if necessary) or under general anaesthetic on a day stay basis.

Dental extractions

The extraction of a tooth is probably the most commonly performed surgical procedure and is often associated with understandable apprehension by the patient. A thorough knowledge of dental anatomy is essential. Most extractions are simple and uncomplicated providing the operator is skilled and the correct technique is followed with the use of the appropriate extraction forceps. A number of factors need to be taken into account:

■ The age of the patient. Extractions in children are generally easy from a technical aspect but may be problematic in terms of patient co-operation. Bone becomes more dense with advancing years and the teeth more brittle, leading to a tendency for teeth to break during extraction.
■ Root filled teeth tend to be more brittle and liable to fracture.
■ The presence of acute infection such as an abscess may sometimes preclude extraction under local analgesia.
■ Medical history: it is important to take into account conditions such as a bleeding diathesis, allergy, diabetes, cardiac or autoimmune

problems. It is also important to ascertain whether the patient is taking any current medication, e.g. steroids, insulin, anticoagulants, etc.

Indications

- Decayed teeth that are beyond repair
- Abscessed teeth that are beyond repair
- Teeth with severe periodontal disease
- Malpositioned teeth preventing orthodontic treatment or denture or bridge construction
- Elective removal of healthy teeth to create space for orthodontic treatment

Diagnosis

Decayed or abscessed teeth are often painful. If the tooth is vital with an intact nerve supply then stimulation with extremes of temperature will generally induce pain. Vitality of a tooth can also be tested by the use of an electric pulp tester. If the tooth is non-vital and abscessed it will usually be tender to pressure either from biting or tapping the tooth.

An abscessed tooth may present with facial swelling. Infection above an upper canine tooth may present with a swollen lower eyelid. Lower premolars and molars may present with swelling in the neck. Upper anterior teeth may cause swelling of the upper lip and lower anterior teeth swelling beneath the chin. Infection of upper lateral incisors occasionally presents with swelling in the palate. If an abscess is treated with antibiotic without extraction then the problem may become chronic and lead to the development of a sinus discharging through the gum or occasionally the skin.

Radiographic examination is essential in order that the root configuration can be assessed. Usually upper anterior teeth and upper second pre-molar teeth will have single roots, as will lower anterior teeth and both lower pre-molars. Upper first pre-molar teeth will usually have two roots and upper first and second molars three roots. Lower first and second molars have two roots.

Aims

Removal of teeth without damage to adjacent teeth or unnecessary removal of adjacent bone.

Pre-operative preparation of the patient

- An explanation of what is involved and informed consent.
- It is important that the surgeon and nurse create an atmosphere of calm and reassurance for the patient.

- If for general anaesthesia, complete standard check list.
- Pre-operative analgesia, e.g. aspirin or paracetamol.

Procedure

Most routine dental extractions are performed under local anaesthesia. More complicated extractions or multiple extractions may necessitate a general anaesthetic. The procedure should be explained to the patient with reassurance that the extraction will be painless. If the extraction is to be undertaken under local anaesthesia then the patient should not be starved. For routine extraction in an adult it is not necessary that the patient be accompanied unless intravenous sedation or general anaesthesia is to be used.

Instruments required

- Oral surgical set with modifications as required (*see* Fig. 4.5)
- Extraction forceps as required (*see* Fig. 4.8)
- Suction
- High density lighting

Anaesthesia

Simple extractions of non-impacted or buried teeth rarely warrant general anaesthesia unless the teeth to be removed are in young children, abscessed or multiple.

General anaesthesia

The patient should have been pre-assessed from a medical point of view. From the nursing perspective there is very little difference in instrumentation or procedure

Local anaesthesia

Many local anaesthetic agents contain a vasoconstrictor such as adrenaline. This is useful in terms of reducing local haemorrhage but it is important that there are no medical contra-indications such as patients with cardiac arrhythmias. Felypressin is an alternative vasoconstrictor. In nervous patients a topical anaesthetic gel can be applied to the injection site. Modem disposable needles are very fine and a local infiltration can be given with very little discomfort. An injection of local anaesthetic is more comfortable for the patient if the cartridge is warmed to body temperature and injected slowly.

Positioning

If the procedure is performed under general anaesthetic in a hospital environment the patient will be supine with a naso-tracheal tube in place to deliver the anaesthetic and the throat will be packed off by the anaesthetist. For very simple extractions, especially in fit children, ambulatory general anaesthetic is still administered.

Under local analgesia the patient should be in a reclining position in a dental chair in such a way that patient and operator are comfortable. The chair should be fully adjustable for both height and recline angle. Should a patient faint during the procedure then there should be a rapid release facility to allow the chair to become fully reclined. Oxygen should be available through a face mask delivery system.

Preparation of operative site

■ Standard peri-oral

Operative procedure

■ The pharynx will be packed off if a general anaesthetic is administered.
■ Under local anaesthetic a light oral gauze pack may be inserted in the mouth in such a way that the patient does not retch.
■ Appropriate local anaesthetic is given.
■ The periodontal ligament space of the tooth to be removed is widened and the tooth subluxed using a straight Coupland's elevator, a periotome or merely by driving the forceps blades along the root of the tooth.
■ During the extraction the patient's head is firmly supported by an assistant or nurse, especially when upper teeth are being extracted.
■ The operator will apply bucco-palatal or bucco-lingual support with thumb and index finger during the extraction manoeuvre.
■ The following teeth are usually single rooted and removal is facilitated by a rotation movement of the forceps:
  □ upper and lower incisor teeth
  □ upper and lower canine teeth
  □ lower pre-molar teeth
■ Upper first pre-molar teeth usually have buccal and palatal roots and are best removed by employing a bucco-palatal movement with the forceps followed by a vertical pull in a downward direction.
■ Upper molars usually have two buccal roots and a larger palatal root. Special forceps are designed to be used on either the right or the left side with beaks that engage the buccal bifurcation. A strong upward movement is followed by firm pressure in a buccal direction to facilitate removal.

- Lower molars are removed by applying the appropriate forceps and exerting extraction force in a buccal direction.
- Upper and lower third molar extractions are considered under the section covering impacted teeth.

Following extraction the edges of the socket are firmly compressed by finger pressure and a sterile pack is applied. The patient can then apply pressure by biting firmly on the pack.

If there appears to be excessive bleeding from the socket then the socket should be sutured. A horizontal mattress suture will effectively prevent soft tissue bleeding in most situations. Occasionally haemorrhage is encountered from the bony socket and it is necessary to insert a sterile packing material into the socket itself. This may be resorbable material or alternatively a small length of ribbon gauze pack impregnated with a suitable material such as Whiteheads varnish. Such a pack will need to be removed at about one week.

A wide range of suture material is available and choice depends upon the clinical circumstances and operator preference. If a strong suture is required then black silk or nylon is appropriate, but both need to be removed. Synthetic resorbable sutures are effective, but can remain for several weeks and be detrimental to oral hygiene. Modern catgut sutures combine reasonable strength and a suitable biodegradation cycle and are good universal sutures in most situations. Sutures should not be cut too short.

Recovery

In the out-patient clinic situation the patient should be made comfortable and detained for 10 minutes with a gauze pressure pack in place. The patient can then be discharged with written post-operative instructions (*see* Information leaflet No 2).

Following general anaesthesia the usual post-operative care routine will be followed. The patient will then be discharged in the care of a responsible adult (*see* Information leaflet No 5).

Post-operative care and follow-up

- Routine uncomplicated extractions should not be associated with any great degree of pain or swelling. Ordinary analgesics such as aspirin or paracetamol should suffice to control post-extraction discomfort.
- The use of warm saline mouth washes encourages healing and maintains good oral hygiene.
- For routine extractions when no bone has been exposed or removed it is generally not necessary to prescribe an antibiotic unless there is a medical indication.

■ In the absence of complications a routine follow-up appointment is not indicated unless non-resorbable sutures have been employed.

Complications

Fracture of the tooth
Not infrequently a root or roots break during an extraction. If the retained root is very small and therefore deeply placed and not associated with any periapical pathology then it is acceptable to leave the fragment *in situ*, having informed the patient. If the root fragment is large or associated with infection, then it should be removed and this will involve surgical exposure and removal which is covered in the next section.

Fracture of the surrounding bone
Frequently pieces of buccal bone fracture. Any loose fragment should be removed and the adjacent edges smoothed and the site should be sutured. Sometimes the extraction of an upper molar can result in fracture of the alveolar bone including the maxillary tuberosity. This is especially likely when teeth become ankylosed with the bone in older patients.

Fracture of the mandible during the removal of a tooth with dental forceps
This is very rare unless there is an unexpected pathology such as a large cyst or tumour. Any such pathology should have been obvious on the pre-operative radiograph.

Displacement of a tooth or root
If a tooth or part of a tooth suddenly disappears it is most important that its whereabouts is identified:

■ The patient should not be alarmed
■ The patient, operator and nurse should make minimal movement
■ The mouth must be thoroughly searched
■ A root fragment may have been sucked into the suction apparatus
■ The tooth or root may have been displaced into the maxillary sinus or the lateral pharyngeal space
■ The tooth or root may have been swallowed
■ The tooth or root may have been inhaled

X-rays may be necessary to confirm the site of the displaced root or tooth. If it cannot be identified within the oro-facial region then a chest X-ray is mandatory.

Oro-antral fistula
The apices of upper pre-molar and molar teeth are intimately related to the maxillary sinus. Following extraction of these teeth a fistula – an opening between the mouth and the sinus – can develop. Predisposing factors leading to a fistula are:

■ Apical abscess
■ Pre-existing sinus disease
■ A traumatic extraction with removal of adjacent bone
■ Fracture of a root with displacement of the fragment into the sinus
■ Displacement of a tooth into the sinus

The management of an oro-antral fistula is covered in a later section.

Damage to adjacent teeth
Teeth adjacent to the tooth to be extracted may be damaged by:

■ The forceps slipping off the tooth
■ The wrong forceps being applied
■ Excessive force with an elevator

Anterior teeth, especially if crowned, are at particular risk when an extraction is performed under general anaesthesia. The anaesthetist will usually employ a laryngoscope during intubation, or to check the position of a naso-tracheal tube. The laryngoscope is metal and may contact the upper incisor teeth during use.

Extraction of the wrong tooth
It is disastrous to extract the wrong tooth, but this can occur when it has been arranged to extract a deciduous tooth which has subsequently been lost naturally, or the X-ray has been wrongly labelled. The rules must be:

■ Check the notes
■ Check the patient
■ Check the X-ray (the presence of fillings is a good method of ensuring the X-ray is correctly orientated)

Infection of socket
'Dry socket' – osteitis of a socket resulting from loss of the blood clot – usually occurs 2 to 4 days after extraction. It is very painful and is more likely to occur following traumatic or difficult extractions, especially with lower pre-molars or molars. The socket should be irrigated with normal saline and packed with a suitable material to relieve symptoms. The incidence of dry socket is reduced with the administration of an antibiotic, especially if the operative procedure is traumatic or if the patient has a

systemic condition predisposing to infection, e.g. diabetes or taking steroid medication.

Pain and swelling
Pain and swelling should not be a feature of a routine successful extraction. Minor discomfort should be managed by analgesics.

Removal of buried roots

Indications

- A root fractured during a dental extraction
- A root associated with periapical pathology
- A root preventing orthodontic treatment
- A root interfering with the fit of a denture
- A root causing painful symptoms
- A root in a patient at special risk from infection, e.g. immuno-compromised or at risk of bacterial endocarditis

If small root fragments are buried and asymptomatic then they do not need to be removed. If a tiny fragment (less than 3 mm in diameter) of root is fractured during extraction of a tooth, attempted retrieval may well cause far more problems for the patient than leaving the fragment *in situ*. The patient must be informed and reassured.

Diagnosis

The position of the buried root may be indicated by symptoms or signs, for example pain under a denture. A root associated with a chronic abscess may well present with a sinus tract discharging pus with an associated pyogenic granuloma at the sinus opening.

X-rays are essential to establish the exact position of the root, the relationship of the adjacent structures and to assess the likely difficulty of surgical removal.

Aim

To remove the root without damage to adjacent structures, for example teeth, nerves or maxillary sinus.

Pre-operative preparation of the patient

- An explanation of what is involved and informed consent
- Standard pre-operative assessment if the procedure is to be done under general anaesthetic

Procedure

Instruments required

- Oral surgical set (*see* Fig. 4.5)
- Oral surgical drill and irrigation delivery system (*see* Fig. 4.14)

Anaesthesia

Local or general.

Positioning

Standard for clinic or operating theatre.

Preparation

- Standard peri-oral
- Oral analgesic if under local anaesthesia, for example aspirin or paracetamol

Operative procedure

The key to successful surgery is adequate access to the surgical site and a clear blood-free surgical field. The nurse has a vital role to play in relation to effective retraction of tissues and in the skilled use of a suction probe in keeping the surgical field free of debris.

Design of the mucoperiosteal flap to achieve access depends upon the position of the buried root or roots and the example given is for the removal of a lower premolar root.

- A two-sided mucoperiosteal flap involving gingival margin and angled extension is raised (Fig. 5.1). In this example care must be taken to avoid damage to the mental nerve.
- Buccal bone is removed with either a chisel or saline cooled drill to

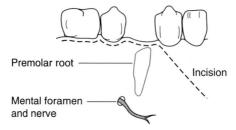

Fig. 5.1   Two-sided flap for removal of a lower premolar root.

expose the root. The use of a chisel under local anaesthesia is limited as even with adequate analgesia the experience is unpleasant for the patient.

■ Once the maximum diameter of the root is exposed an appropriate elevator is insinuated between bone and root and the root is subluxed by a twisting or rotating movement.

■ Following removal of the root the socket should be gently curetted and irrigated with normal saline.

■ The flap is then accurately repositioned and sutured in place.

Post-operative care and follow-up

■ More swelling, though not necessarily more discomfort, might be expected than following a simple extraction. Post operative symptoms depend upon the size of the flap raised, the amount of bone removed and the length of the procedure.

■ Antibiotics and analgesics should be prescribed.

■ Standard post-operative instructions should be given in written form (*see* Information leaflets No 2 and No 5).

■ A review appointment is generally appropriate, especially if a non-resorbable suture has been used.

Complications

■ Wound infection

■ Damage to adjacent structures especially teeth and nerves

■ Excessive traction applied to a flap in the lower pre-molar area can cause prolonged paraesthesia of the mental nerve

■ Soft tissue flaps, unless designed and retracted correctly, are particularly susceptible to damage by a bur

■ Vertical force to upper molar roots can cause them to be displaced into the maxillary sinus

Removal of impacted and ectopic teeth, odontomes and supernumerary teeth

It is very common for teeth to develop normally but fail to erupt into the correct position in the dental arch. Impaction implies that a tooth cannot erupt into its normal position. The size of the teeth and the size and shape of the jaws are genetically determined. If an individual inherits a small jaw from one parent and large teeth from the other then crowding and impaction of teeth is likely. Third molars are the most likely to become impacted, followed by pre-molars and upper canine teeth.

Odontomes are benign disorganised overgrowths of dental tissues resulting in a calcified mass which may displace or obstruct the eruption of adjacent teeth.

Supernumerary teeth can occur anywhere in the dental arches and represent extra teeth which may be anatomically normal, though usually smaller, but can be rudimentary or malformed. A common site is in the midline between the upper anterior teeth where the supernumerary tooth (mesiodens) may impede the normal eruption of the permanent incisor teeth.

The principles which govern the successful removal of impacted teeth are:

- Adequate pre-operative assessment
- Adequate exposure
- Gentle handling of the tissues
- Adequate removal of bone
- Division of the tooth if indicated
- Thorough curettage and irrigation of the socket
- Accurate re-positioning of the flap
- Good pre- and post-operative patient information and communication

Indications for removal

The removal of impacted teeth, odontomes and supernumerary teeth is a surgical procedure usually involving removal of adjacent bone. In many cases local anaesthesia with intravenous sedation or general anaesthesia is indicated. If the impacted teeth are lying deeply and there are no clinical or radiological features suggesting an active pathology then removal is not indicated. Removal of impacted teeth is a procedure not without risk in terms of damaging adjacent structures such as teeth and nerves. Surgical intervention is indicated:

- When there is repeated infection
- If the impaction is causing decay in an adjacent tooth
- If there is change in the surrounding bone on X-ray examination, e.g. cyst formation
- If the impaction is preventing planned orthodontic treatment

Diagnosis

Impacted teeth may be asymptomatic. Symptoms and signs of infection are commonly presented with:

- Pain and tenderness
- Bad taste
- Food packing

- Facial swelling
- Swollen lymph glands
- Limitation of opening
- Systemic upset

The assessment and surgical treatment of impacted and supernumerary teeth and odontomes is essentially similar and involves common principles:

- Sex, age and build of patient; dense bone will influence treatment planning
- Medical history including medication
- Patient co-operation in relation to the anticipated difficulty of surgery
- Anaesthetic – local, local with intravenous sedation, general anaesthesia

Radiological examination and assessment

X-rays are essential to determine the position of the tooth, the root configuration, changes in adjacent structures and proximity of important structures such as the inferior dental canal, the mental nerve and the maxillary sinus. A very good screening X-ray is the orthopantomograph (OPT) which on one X-ray film shows both jaws and all the teeth. However it is sometimes important to obtain a high definition picture of the individual tooth to be removed and this can be effected by an intra-oral periapical X-ray and/or a standard occlusal view.

Lower third molar teeth

The difficulty of surgery relates to the type and depth of impaction. The deeper the tooth the more difficult the access and the more bone required to be removed and the greater he danger of damaging adjacent structures.

Type of impaction (Fig. 5.2)

- Mesioangular
- Horizontal
- Vertical
- Distoangular

Root pattern

- Wisdom teeth may be single or multirooted and the roots may be conical or curved.
- Long roots increase the difficulty of removal and are more common in some ethnic groups.

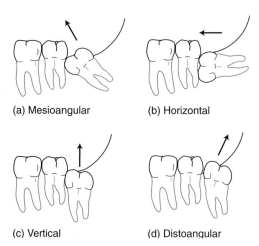

(a) Mesioangular   (b) Horizontal

(c) Vertical   (d) Distoangular

Fig. 5.2   Classification of lower impacted third molar teeth.

- Roots may involve and even embrace the inferior dental canal. Under such circumstances the tooth and roots must be carefully divided and removed in sections to avoid damage to the inferior dental nerve leading to possible permanent numbness of the ipsilateral mandibular teeth and lip.
- The root pattern of the adjacent second molar is important. If it is conical, inappropriate application of an elevator to a wisdom tooth can lead to elevation of the second molar rather than the wisdom tooth.
- Careless application of an elevator can dislodge a distal filling in the second molar, especially if the restoration is overhanging.

Upper third molar teeth

An OPT X-ray is generally sufficient in terms of assessing surgical difficulty. Highly placed upper third molar teeth are at risk of being displaced into the maxillary sinus or into the adjacent soft tissues and should not be removed unless there is a definite clinical indication.

Pre-molar teeth

An OPT X-ray and often a periapical X-ray are indicated. It is sometimes necessary to divide pre-molar teeth as there may be insufficient space to elevate them piecemeal. It is very important to avoid damaging adjacent teeth and, in the case of mandibular pre-molars, the mental nerve as it leaves the mental foramen.

Canine teeth

Upper canine teeth may be impacted buccally, in the line of the dental arch or palatally. A combination of an OPT and a lateral cephalometric X-ray or two periapical X-rays at different angles with an upper occlusal X-ray will generally facilitate an accurate assessment of the position of the tooth. Lower canine teeth are less frequently impacted and are usually palpable.

Odontomes and supernumerary teeth

These will often present as an incidental X-ray finding with no clinical symptoms and should be assessed with the aid of intra-oral periapical X-rays

Removal of lower third molar teeth

Aims

Removal of the impacted tooth without damage to the adjacent structures.

Pre-operative preparation of the patient

- Explanation, and informed consent with specific reference to sensory disturbance of the lower lip or tongue (Information leaflet No 7)
- Standard pre-operative assessment if the procedure is to be done under general anaesthetic

Procedure

The example given is the removal of a lower wisdom tooth which has a mesioangular impaction.

Instruments required

- Oral surgical set (*see* Fig. 4.5)
- Oral surgical drill with burs and irrigation delivery system (*see* Fig. 4.14)

Anaesthesia

Local anaesthesia with or without intravenous sedation or general anaesthesia.

PATIENT INFORMATION LEAFLET No 7

ORAL and MAXILLOFACIAL SURGERY DEPARTMENT

REMOVAL OF IMPACTED WISDOM TEETH

1. There are various reasons for removing impacted wisdom teeth, but the most common is related to recurrent infection when the teeth cannot erupt properly because there is insufficient room at the back of the mouth.
2. The procedure is carried out either under local anaesthetic (an injection to completely numb the tooth and the area around it) as an out-patient, or under general anaesthetic (being asleep) which involves coming into hospital, but not usually needing to stay overnight.
3. The procedure normally involves the gum being cut to uncover the tooth. Bone may have to be removed from around the tooth (usually with a drill) and the wisdom tooth may need to be divided into several separate pieces. The gum is stitched back into position at the end of the procedure using stitches which normally fall out themselves.
4. After wisdom teeth have been removed there will be some discomfort and some swelling and stiffness will probably develop over the next 24 hours.
5. Numbness of the lower lip or tongue can occur after the removal of lower wisdom teeth. This is because the nerves giving the feeling in the lip or tongue run very close to the wisdom teeth. If this occurs it is almost always temporary (but may last several months). Very occasionally, however, the effects can be permanent.
6. The pain is controlled by painkillers such as paracetamol or ibuprofen, or one that has been prescribed before leaving hospital.
7. A course of antibiotics is also prescribed to prevent infection.
8. It is very important to keep the mouth as clean as possible to prevent infection and promote rapid healing. Normal tooth brushing should be carried out as far as possible, but in the wound area use mouthbaths (hot saline or bicarbonate) ideally every 3 to 4 hours, but certainly after meals, beginning the day after surgery.
9. You will be given a follow-up appointment for approximately one week after your operation
10. If you have any special problems ring . . . . for advice.

Positioning

Standard for the clinic or operating theatre.

Preparation

- Standard peri-oral
- Oral analgesic if under local anaesthesia

Operative procedure

A soft tissue flap is outlined (Fig. 5.3) and a mucoperiosteal flap raised. The incision is made firmly down to the underlying bone. The initial raising of the flap may be made with the aid of a Warwick-James elevator and then fully developed with a Fickling's and/or Howarth's periosteal elevator. A buccal retractor is inserted to hold the flap in the retracted position. Continuous suction is essential. The lingual mucoperiosteum is carefully elevated and a suitable retractor is inserted to protect the lingual nerve, which has a very close relationship to the inner aspect of the jaw in the lower third molar area. The assistant or nurse should not apply forceful traction to the lingual tissues.

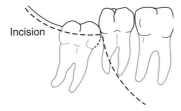

Fig. 5.3 Incision for removal of impacted lower third molar tooth.

Under general anaesthesia a combination of sharp 3 mm and 5 mm chisels may be used for bone removal. Under local analgesia bone removal should be with saline cooled surgical burs. Sufficient bone must be removed to expose the maximum width of the crown of the impacted tooth. Generally (with a bur) a buccal gutter should be developed and then the distal aspect of the tooth relieved. Using a chisel the main area of bone removal is distal and lingual to the tooth. A decision to divide the tooth may have been made on the basis of the pre-operative assessment or during the surgical procedure. Dividing the tooth using a bur or osteotome will usually mean that less bone will need to be removed. During this process the nurse or assistant has a vital role in maintaining a clear operative field by retraction and suction.

After the tooth has been exposed or divided, a suitable elevator – usually a straight Warwick-James or fine Couplands – will be insinuated into a predetermined application point and gently rotated. Once the tooth is subluxed the operator must assess whether elevation and delivery is possible without the need for further bone removal or tooth division. It must be remembered that when a mesioangular impaction is elevated upwards there is a tendency for a curved distal root to move downwards, potentially damaging the inferior dental bundle if it is in intimate proximity to the root. In such a case X-ray pre-assessment would indicate that tooth division rather than elevation as a whole is the procedure of choice in such a situation.

Following removal the tooth must be inspected to ensure that no root fracture has occurred. The socket is irrigated and any remnants of dental follicle or fragments of bone should be removed. Once it has been ensured that there is no continuing haemorrhage from the socket the flap is replaced and sutured. Choice of suture material depends on operator personal preference, but a soft resorbable suture is best for the patient. Accurate re-positioning of the flap is important to minimise healing problems. Usually two or three sutures are adequate

Post-operative care and follow up

- Some discomfort and swelling is inevitable following third molar surgery when bone has been removed and adequate analgesia must be provided. The post-operative course will be smoother if an adequate explanation of what is to be expected is given to the patient in written form (*see* Information leaflets No 2 and No 5).
- Antibiotics should be prescribed when bone has been removed or when infection is obvious at the time of surgery.
- A vigorous oral hygiene regime should be started the day following surgery, e.g. warm saline or chlorhexidine mouth baths four times daily.
- In most instances one post-operative out-patient review will be appropriate to ensure there are no complications.

Complications

- Fracture of root(s)
- Displacement of root(s)
- Fracture of mandible
- Infection
- Haemorrhage
- Damage to the inferior dental nerve
- Damage to the lingual nerve

The most important complication is damage to the adjacent nerves. Damage to the inferior dental nerve and lingual nerve can be caused by direct trauma from a bur or chisel or through compression by a root during elevation. Damage to the lingual nerve can also result through excessive retraction on the lingual tissues by an assistant. Nerve damage is usually temporary but can be permanent.

Removal of upper third molar teeth

The same general principles apply in relation to the removal of impacted upper wisdom teeth. The buccal bone is much thinner and can often be removed by hand chiselling rather than using a bur. (An example of a flap is shown in Fig. 5.4.)

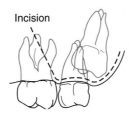

Fig. 5.4 Incision for removal of impacted upper third molar tooth.

Complications

- Fracture of the maxillary tuberosity
- Displacement of the tooth or a root into the soft tissues or maxillary antrum
- Oro-antral fistula
- Damage to the adjacent second molar

Removal of upper canine teeth

Palpable buccally placed canine teeth can usually be approached by a simple linear incision over the crown (Fig. 5.5). The very thin layer of bone can be removed by hand chiselling. More commonly upper canine teeth are impacted in the palate and approached by a palatal flap (Fig. 5.6). A general anaesthetic is often indicated, especially in younger patients. General anaesthesia permits the use of a chisel to remove bone to uncover the tooth. Especial care is necessary to elevate the tooth without causing damage to adjacent incisor or premolar roots. It is sometimes necessary to section the tooth with a surgical bur. The flap is approximated with resorbable sutures.

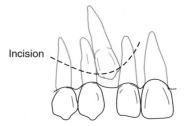

Fig. 5.5   Incision for removal of a labially placed impacted upper canine tooth.

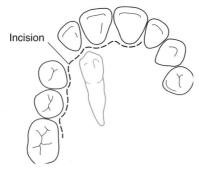

Fig. 5.6   Incision for removal of a palatally placed impacted upper canine tooth.

Removal of supernumerary teeth

Supernumerary teeth in the anterior maxilla may need to be removed if they are preventing the normal eruption of the permanent incisors. A palatal flap is used and palatal bone removed to uncover the super-numerary tooth or teeth. Great care is necessary to identify and avoid damage to any developing and unerupted upper incisor teeth.

Surgical uncovering of unerupted teeth

This is undertaken to allow eruption and orthodontic repositioning of the unerupted tooth into its correct position in the dental arch. The unerupted upper canine tooth is most frequently involved. If the tooth is located in the palate, a palatal flap is raised and bone removed in the same way as for removal of the tooth except that only the crown of the tooth is uncovered, taking great care that the tooth is not damaged in the process. Following this a 'window' is cut in the palatal flap overlying the crown of the tooth and the flap repositioned (Fig. 5.7). A pack of ribbon gauze soaked in Whitehead's varnish is sutured over the mucosal defect to act as a dressing and inhibit regrowth of the flap over the defect. A dental plate

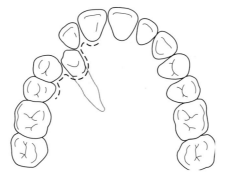

Fig. 5.7 Crown of impacted canine uncovered by excision of palatal mucoperiosteum.

and suitable dressing may be used instead of a pack. An orthodontic bracket may be fixed to the tooth during the procedure. If a pack is used it is removed at 1 to 2 weeks after surgery.

For upper canines which are unerupted but on the labial aspect of the dental arch, a flap is raised and the tooth uncovered. No mucosa is excised and the flap simply repositioned at a superior level to leave the crown of the tooth exposed (Fig. 5.8). A pack is generally not necessary with this procedure.

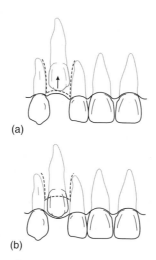

(a)

(b)

Fig. 5.8 Crown of impacted canine uncovered by raising a labial mucoperiosteal flap and suturing at a higher level.

Transplantation of teeth

Unerupted teeth may be transplanted if orthodontic repositioning is not feasible or desirable. Upper canine teeth are most frequently involved. The tooth is removed as atraumatically as possible using a suitable flap, and stored in normal saline. A socket is prepared in the alveolar bone using large conical burs, and the tooth fixed into position using a dental splint for approximately 6 weeks.

In the short term most transplanted teeth perform satisfactorily, but a proportion suffer from root resorption and have a poorer long term prognosis.

Oro-antral fistula

The maxillary sinus is intimately related to the upper pre-molar and molar teeth. Extraction of these teeth can result in a communication between the mouth and the sinus. If the extraction is uncomplicated and there is no sinus disease then any small communication is usually sealed by a blood clot and normal healing occurs. If, however, a larger defect occurs or there is pre-existing sinus or tooth infection then a fistula may develop. A fistula is an epithelial lined tract between the mouth and the sinus and once established will not close without surgical intervention. Fracture of part of a root with subsequent displacement into the maxillary sinus will also predispose to fistula formation.

If, following an extraction, a communication between the sinus and the mouth is suspected the socket is sutured, an antibiotic prescribed and the patient advised not to blow the nose. If a large or obvious defect is noted between the mouth and the sinus at the time of extraction it is reasonable to attempt primary repair and closure, but this is usually carried out as a secondary procedure. It should be remembered that occasionally an oro-antral fistula can present as a result of antral disease such as a tumour destroying the bone and ulcerating through into the mouth.

Diagnosis

If, after 3 to 4 weeks have elapsed, any of the following features are present then a fistula has developed:

- Air escape into the mouth on raising intra-nasal pressure, e.g. blowing the nose
- A salty taste
- Reflux of fluids into the nasal cavity when drinking
- Prolapse of the antral lining into the mouth
- Difficulty on drawing on a cigarette if the patient is a smoker

Sometimes development of a fistula may be associated with an acute infection of the maxillary sinus leading to pus formation in the antrum and considerable pain. X-ray examination of the sinus may reveal an opaque maxillary antrum or a fluid level.

Aims

- To eliminate infection
- To close the fistula

Pre-operative preparation of the patient

- Patient information and informed consent.
- Usually closure of an oro-antral fistula will be under a general anaesthetic and the usual pre-operative assessment will apply.

Procedure

A buccal advancement flap is most commonly used

Instruments required

- Oral surgical set (*see* Fig. 4.5)
- Caldwell-Luc and nasal antrostomy set

Anaesthesia

A general anaesthetic is usually given.

Positioning

Standard positioning with a naso-tracheal tube in place on the opposite side to the fistula.

Preparation of operative site

Standard peri-oral preparation.

Operative procedure

- The fistula is probed to assess the extent of the underlying defect, and the fistula then excised and a mucoperiosteal flap is raised (Fig. 5.9(a)). The bony defect will now be visible (Fig. 5.9(b)).
- The maxillary sinus is irrigated and cleared of granulations and polyps and this may be possible through the bony defect if this is large.

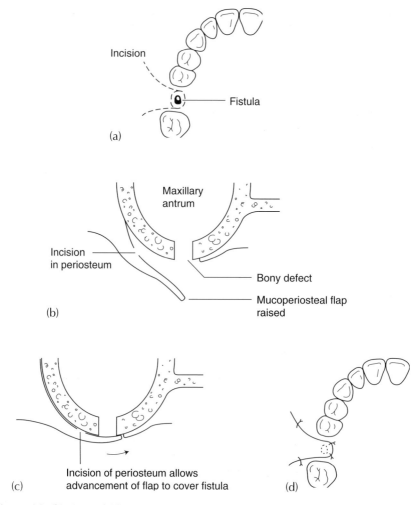

Fig. 5.9(a), (b), (c) and (d)   Closure of oro-antral fistula.

- Sometimes a Caldwell–Luc approach to the sinus via a modified flap allows better access. If a root or tooth has been previously displaced into the sinus the extended access will allow easier retrieval.
- The flap is advanced to cover the defect without tension by incising the periosteum on the undersurface of the flap (Fig. 5.9(c)).
- The flap is sutured using either 4-0 synthetic resorbable or non-resorbable sutures (Fig. 5.9(d)). It is preferable to employ some vertical mattress sutures so that the edge of the flap is slightly everted. To facilitate this, three sutures are inserted but not tied until all are in place. The nurse or assistant clamps the suture ends with a mosquito forceps until all three sutures are ready to be tied.

■ If the sinus has been infected it may be necessary to perform a nasal antrostomy and insert a drain from the sinus to the exterior via the nostril.

Post-operative care and follow-up

■ The patient must avoid nose blowing
■ Antibiotics must be prescribed
■ A nasal decongestant may be prescribed
■ Warm saline mouth washes four times daily
■ Out-patient review at 7 to 10 days for suture removal if resorbable sutures have not been employed

Complications

Wound breakdown is possible, with recurrence of fistula. If the flap has been correctly positioned without tension and post-operative instructions carefully followed then breakdown is not common as the blood supply to the area is very good.

Alternative method of closure

A flap of palatal mucosa based on the greater palatine artery is less frequently employed as it is technically more difficult and morbidity for the patient is greater. The indications for use are:

■ Inadequate buccal tissue for an advancement flap
■ The fistula is sited on the palatal aspect of the alveolus
■ Failure of a buccal advancement flap

Anaesthesia, positioning and preparation are as for the buccal advancement flap. The fistula is excised as previously described and sinus lavage is performed. A 'finger' of palatal tissue is incised down to the palatal bone and elevated. The flap is rotated over the fistula defect and sutured as previously described (Fig. 5.10). The bare area in the palate can be covered with a dressing of half inch ribbon gauze soaked in Whitehead's varnish and retained by two or three black silk sutures. The donor area granulates and re-epithelialises. Although the flap tends to shrink and flatten there is often some residual bulkiness which can cause a problem in relation to later denture construction.

Post-operative care is essentially the same as with a buccal advancement flap. Breakdown of the flap is rare, but should it occur then there would need to be recourse to a more complex method of closure such as a tongue flap or island flap.

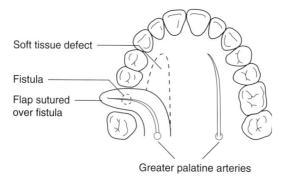

Fig. 5.10   Closure of oro-antral fistula with palatal flap.

Cysts and periapical lesions

Jaw cysts are common and originate from epithelium remaining in the tissue following tooth formation (and for this reason are termed odontogenic). The cause of the proliferation of the epithelial cells to form a cyst is not fully understood, but in the commonest type of cyst (apical or radicular), epithelial growth is triggered by the stimulus of a periapical granuloma, which in turn is caused by pulpal necrosis within a tooth (*see* Fig. 5.12(a)).

Other types of cyst related to tooth formation are the dentigerous cyst and the keratocyst. A dentigerous cyst arises when cystic change takes place in the follicle or sac surrounding a developing tooth. Most commonly affected are the lower third molars (*see* Fig. 5.11). A keratocyst is a less common jaw cyst characterised by a keratinising epithelial lining. Keratocysts have a greater tendency to recur than other jaw cysts.

Non-odontogenic cysts are relatively rare. The incisive canal (nasopalatine) cyst arises in the upper jaw from epithelial remnants of the nasopalatine duct which connects the oral and nasal cavities in the embryo.

Jaw cysts grow slowly, and initially without symptoms. Eventually they may cause swelling and deformity. Pain is usually related to infection. Adjacent structures may be involved – in the upper jaw, the nasal cavity and maxillary sinus, and in the lower jaw the neurovascular canal. Eventually the jaw may be significantly weakened.

Treatment of all jaw cysts is principally enucleation. Marsupialisation (surgical de-roofing) may occasionally be appropriate for some very large cysts to allow bony regeneration and reduce the risk of damage to adjacent structures during enucleation.

Surgery for jaw cysts

Examples are given of the procedures for two common types of cyst.

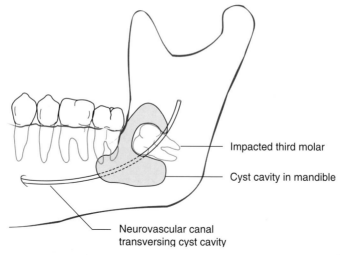

Impacted third molar

Cyst cavity in mandible

Neurovascular canal
transversing cyst cavity

Fig. 5.11   Dentigerous cyst.

Enucleation of a dentigerous cyst

Related to an unerupted lower third molar tooth, (Fig. 5.11).

Indications

■ Cyst formation in relation to a developing or unerupted tooth

Diagnosis

■ May be asymptomatic
■ Swelling and pain
■ Radiographs essential

Aims

Elimination of pathology without damage to adjacent structures, in this case the neurovascular canal and its contents, and adjacent teeth.

Pre-operative preparation of the patient

■ Patient information and informed consent with special reference to sensory disturbance of the lower lip and possible loss of related teeth. With very large cysts there may be some risk of fracture of the mandible during the procedure or post-operatively.
■ If for general anaesthesia, complete the standard check list.

Procedure

Instruments required

- Oral surgical set (*see* Fig. 4.5)
- Oral surgical drill with irrigation (*see* Fig. 4.14)

Anaesthesia

Usually general.

Positioning

Standard for the operating theatre.

Preparation

Standard peri-oral preparation.

Operative procedure

- A soft tissue flap is outlined and a single layer mucoperiosteal flap is raised to expose the bone overlying the cyst
- Bone is removed using a drill or chisel to gain access to the cyst cavity
- The cyst lining is stripped from the walls of the cavity and retained for histological examination
- The unerupted third molar is elevated from the cavity after further bone removal
- The cyst cavity is thoroughly irrigated, any remnants of cyst lining removed, and the flap sutured in its original position
- The oral cavity and pharynx are inspected and cleared by suction, and the throat pack removed
- The lips are lubricated with petroleum jelly or steroid ointment

Post-operative care and follow-up

- Standard written post-operative instructions for the procedure (*see* Information leaflets No 2 and No 5).
- Some swelling, stiffness and discomfort will be present for several days.
- Antibiotic, analgesic/anti-inflammatory medication is prescribed.
- Oral hygiene instruction is given.
- Review the appointment after one week.
- Longer term follow-up with radiographs.

Complications

- Wound infection and breakdown.
- Sensory disturbances of the lower lip due to damage to the inferior alveolar nerve which may lie within the cyst cavity.
- Fracture of the mandible.

Enucleation of a maxillary apical cyst

Including an apicectomy and retrograde root filling.

Indications

- Apical cysts or granulomata occur in relation to teeth in which the pulp becomes necrotic, usually due to trauma or dental caries.
- Root filling is the initial treatment for these teeth, but in addition surgical removal of the cyst or granuloma, resection of the root apex (apicectomy) and sealing of the apical root canal (retrograde root filling) may be necessary.

Diagnosis

- May be asymptomatic
- Pain, swelling, tenderness, sinus formation
- Radiographs essential

Aims

- Elimination of pathology without damage to adjacent teeth.

Pre-operative preparation of the patient

- Patient information and informed consent (Information leaflet No 8).
- If for general anaesthesia, complete the standard check list.

Procedure

The example given is for an upper incisor tooth with a small associated cyst (Fig. 5.12(a)). The tooth has previously been root filled and restored by a post crown, making further access to the root canal for re-root filling impossible.

Instruments required

- Surgical set (periapical) (*see* Fig. 4.6)
- Oral surgical drills with straight and contra angle (microhead) handpieces and irrigation system (*see* Fig. 4.14)

PATIENT INFORMATION LEAFLET No 8

ORAL and MAXILLOFACIAL SURGERY DEPARTMENT

APICECTOMY

1. Apicectomy is an operation carried out to remove infection or a cyst from the bone around the end of the root of a tooth.
2. It is usually carried out under local anaesthetic.
3. After local anaesthetic has been given to completely numb the area, the gum is cut and lifted to uncover the area at the end of the root of the tooth.
4. The bone is then drilled, any infected tissue (or the cyst) is removed and the end of the root of the tooth is sealed.
5. The gum is then stitched back into place. The stitches will usually fall out themselves.
6. After the effect of the local anaesthetic has worn off, there will be some discomfort and some swelling will probably develop over the next 24 hours.
7. The pain is controlled by painkillers such as paracetamol or ibuprofen, or one that has been prescribed before leaving hospital.
8. A course of antibiotics is also prescribed to prevent infection.
9. It is very important to keep the mouth as clean as possible to prevent infection and promote rapid healing. Normal tooth brushing should be carried out as far as possible, but in the wound area use mouthbaths (hot saline or bicarbonate) ideally every 3 to 4 hours, but certainly after meals, beginning the day after surgery.
10. You will be given a follow-up appointment for approximately one week after your operation.
11. If you have any special problems ring . . . . for advice.

- Amalgam pluggers and carrier
- Amalgam mixer

Anaesthesia

Local or general.

Positioning

Standard for clinic or operating theatre.

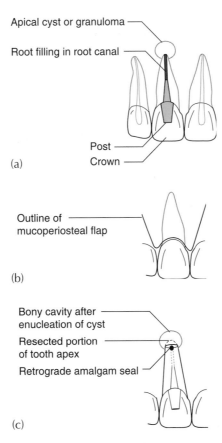

Apical cyst or granuloma

Root filling in root canal

Post

Crown

(a)

Outline of
mucoperiosteal flap

(b)

Bony cavity after
enucleation of cyst

Resected portion
of tooth apex

Retrograde amalgam seal

(c)

Fig. 5.12(a), (b) and (c)   Enucleation of apical cyst, apicectomy and retrograde root filling.

Preparation

Standard peri-oral.

Operative procedure

■ A soft tissue flap is outlined as shown (Fig. 5.12(b)), and a single layer mucoperiosteal flap is raised to expose the bone overlying the cyst. If the cyst or apical pathology is extensive, the flap may be enlarged correspondingly to give good access.

■ Bone is removed with a saline cooled drill to gain access to the cyst cavity, and the cyst lining or granuloma enucleated and retained for histopathological examination.

■ The apex of the tooth root is resected, a small cavity prepared in the resected root face and a seal (amalgam or cement) inserted into the cavity (Fig. 5.12(c)).

- The whole area is thoroughly irrigated with normal saline and the flap sutured into its original position.
- The oral cavity and pharynx are inspected and cleared by suction and the throat pack removed (general anaesthesia).
- The lips are lubricated with petroleum jelly or steroid ointment.

Post-operative care and follow-up

- Standard written post-operative instructions appropriate for the procedure (*see* Information leaflet No 2)
- Some swelling and discomfort will usually be present for several days
- Antibiotics and analgesics will usually be prescribed
- Oral hygiene is important, e.g. warm saline or chlorhexidine mouth baths in the wound area four times daily
- A review appointment after one week when a post-operative radiograph may be taken
- Longer term follow-up and radiographs may be necessary

Complications

- Wound infection and breakdown
- Loss of related tooth or teeth

Drainage of abscesses

Orofacial infection may have several origins, including the skin, salivary glands and lymph nodes, but the teeth remain the commonest source of orofacial abscess formation.

Simple, uncomplicated dentoalveolar abscesses may be drained intra-orally under local anaesthetic by an incision directly over the abscess (Fig. 5.13). More severe infections which may involve the upper airway and become life threatening are managed according to the following principles:

- Admission to hospital for assessment and monitoring
- Systemic antibiotic treatment
- Surgical drainage and removal of the source of the infection

Occasionally infection will settle with antibiotic treatment alone, but if pus is present this must be drained and a general anaesthetic will usually be necessary. The siting of an external skin incision will depend on the location of the collection of pus, and cosmetic considerations, but in general the sequence of events during the procedure is as follows:

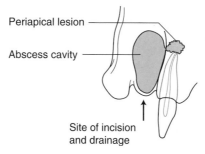

Periapical lesion

Abscess cavity

Site of incision
and drainage

Fig. 5.13 Drainage of abscess.

- Skin incision
- Blunt dissection using mosquito or sinus forceps through the sub-cutaneous tissue to enter the abscess cavity
- Thorough drainage of the abscess cavity, with pus samples taken for microbiological examination
- Drain placed and sutured in position
- Wound dressing

Patient monitoring should continue on the ward and the drain left in place until drainage has ceased.

Summary

Numerically, dentoalveolar procedures account for a large proportion of the case load in the specialty. Most patients are treated under local anaesthetic or day case general anaesthetic. The role of the nurse is paramount and may be summarised as:

- Creation of an optimal environment for pre-operative assessment and information for patients.
- Facilitating the smooth and efficient running of the operating facility.
- Ensuring that measures for post-operative information, after care and follow-up are in place.

6

Benign Soft Tissue Lesions

G. Pell and C. Yates

The purpose of this chapter is to describe the presentation and treatment of the most frequently encountered benign lesions of the oral mucosa. Such lesions are common and may account for 25% of all referrals to departments of oral and maxillofacial surgery. Benign conditions may present as swellings, ulceration, redness, white patches and pigmented areas, although it must be remembered that malignancy may also present in these forms (*see* Chapter 11) and patients may be very anxious about this possibility. On occasions, abnormalities of the oral mucosa may be related to systemic disease especially blood or gastro-intestinal disorders, but these conditions are beyond the scope of this book.

Mucous membrane

The origin of most benign soft tissue lesions of the mouth is the mucous membrane. This is a skin-like structure comprising a surface epithelium and deeper connective tissue layer lining the oral cavity. The lining is modified in certain areas according to function. On the gingivae (gums), hard palate and dorsum of the tongue, a keratinised surface layer gives some protection from the friction produced by mastication.

The keratinised areas of the mouth are paler in colour than the non-keratinised areas (lips, cheeks, floor of the mouth, soft palate and oro-pharynx) where the underlying vascular connective tissue shows through the more transparent epithelium to give the normal red colour of the oral mucous membrane.

In some parts of the mouth (gingivae and parts of the hard palate) the connective tissue of the mucous membrane is attached directly to the underlying bone (a muco-periosteum) producing a tough immobile layer. Elsewhere a submucous layer of connective tissue gives greater mobility and elasticity to the mucous membrane.

Lying beneath the oral mucous membrane (and giving the structure its name) are numerous mucus secreting glands. These are present throughout the mouth, but chiefly inside the lips and cheeks and on the hard and soft palates. The glands secrete a lubricating viscid fluid containing mucin onto the mucous membrane surface.

Mucous cysts (mucous extravasation cysts)
(**see also** Chapter 8)

Clinical appearance and features (Fig. 6.1)

Mucous cysts are generally regarded to be of traumatic origin, and are usually associated with the minor salivary glands in the lower lip. They present as smooth, sessile, soft swellings, varying in size from 2 mm to 2 cm or more in diameter. The colour is typically bluish with a translucent hue when the cyst is superficial, but if more deeply placed, may have a normal mucosal colour. It is unusual to find them in the upper lip, or elsewhere in the mouth, although mucous glands are present throughout

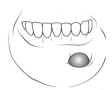

Fig. 6.1   Mucous cyst.

the mouth. There may be a history of trauma to the front of the mouth. Frequently the cyst will vary in size, and occasionally will disappear entirely.

Pathogenesis and histology

The minor salivary glands present throughout the mouth consist of a collection of gland acini, which are connected to the surface of the oral epithelium via a small epithelial lined duct. If the oral mucosa of the lower lip is dried and observed, small beads of mucus will appear on the surface, demonstrating the openings of these small ducts.

The lips are frequently traumatised and it is thought that the epithelial lined duct, conveying the mucus to the surface, is ruptured. The mucus that continues to be produced passes into the tissues through the damaged duct and collects to form a retention cyst. The cyst does not have a lining of epithelial cells, and therefore is not a true cyst. The glandular acini are not damaged and continue to secrete mucus and a point may be reached when the mucosal surface ruptures and the mucoid material is released, with the apparent disappearance of the cyst. When the oral epithelium heals, the mucus begins to collect again, and the cyst recurs.

Treatment

The treatment of these lesions is by excision (*see* Chapter 8, Fig. 8.7) or cryosurgery (*see below*) usually in the out-patient department.

Papilloma (Fig. 6.2)

Clinical appearance

The papilloma is a common benign lesion originating from the surface epithelium of the mouth. It is sometimes confused with the fibroepithelial polyp (*see below*), but it has a distinctive clinical appearance of a small warty like growth, similar to a cauliflower. It is well circumscribed and usually pedunculated and found on the tongue, lips, buccal mucosa, gingivae and palate, particularly the area adjacent to the uvula. It is usually pink in colour, but sometimes may appear white. It usually measures only 2 to 4 mm in diameter, but can attain much larger proportions. It may occur at any age, even in children.

Histology

In appearance it consists of numerous finger like projections extending above the surface of the mucosa. The projections are made up of a con-

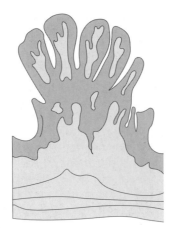

Fig. 6.2   Cross section of papilloma (5 mm in diameter).

tinuous layer of stratified squamous epithelium, supported by a thin core of connective tissue carrying the nutrient blood vessels. In some areas the epithelium may be thickened showing an increase in the keratin layer (hyperkeratosis), giving the lesion its white appearance.

Treatment

Surgical excision is the treatment of choice, and the excision biopsy should include the complete stalk and the adjacent part of the connective tissue. Histological examination of the excised specimen is essential.

Fibroepithelial polyp (Fig. 6.3)

Clinical appearance

The fibroepithelial polyp is a very common, slowly growing lesion found in the mouth. It may occur at any age, but is common in the third, fourth and fifth decades. The fibroepithelial polyp may appear anywhere in the mouth, and is usually the result of irritation or trauma. It is therefore very commonly seen in the buccal mucosa adjacent to the occlusal line of the cheek teeth. It has a smooth surface, but occasionally is roughened, giving it the appearance of a papilloma. These lesions can vary in shape and size from a few millimetres to 1 to 2 cm in diameter, and are attached to the mucosa on a broad base (sessile) or by a stalk (pedunculated). When they arise in the hard palate under a denture, they appear flattened (leaf fibroma). On the gingivae the term fibrous epulis is used.

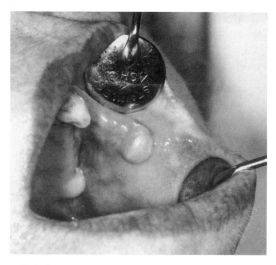

Fig. 6.3 Fibroepithelial polyp in the cheek.

Histology

Histologically the lesion consists of hyperplastic connective tissue covered by stratified squamous epithelium.

Treatment

The treatment of choice is surgical excision under local anaesthesia, together with a small part of its base. It rarely recurs.

Pyogenic granuloma (Fig. 6.4)

Aetiology

The pyogenic granuloma arises as a result of minor chronic trauma to the tissues, and non-specific infection. It may be seen following a tooth extraction, where bone debris has not been removed, from the sharp edge of a subgingival cavity or from the irritation of subgingival calculus. Poor oral hygiene is often a contributory factor.

Clinical appearance

This lesion most commonly arises on the gingiva, but may also appear on the lips, tongue and buccal mucosa. It presents as a pedunculated or sessile swelling, whose surface can be smooth or warty in appearance, and has a reddish or purplish colour, depending on its vascularity. The

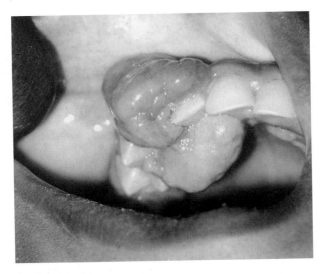

Fig. 6.4 Pyogenic granuloma.

granuloma develops rapidly, and then remains static for a period of time. It bleeds readily to touch.

Histology

The lesion is very vascular, and contains numerous vascular channels and fibroblasts. There is also a fairly dense collection of chronic inflammatory cells. A thin and atrophic layer of oral epithelium covers the surface of the lesion, which may show areas of ulceration. If left untreated, the lesion tends to lose its vascularity and becomes more fibrous in nature.

A lesion very similar to the pyogenic granuloma and occurring in pregnant women is the 'pregnancy tumour' (Fig. 6.5). Histologically, this is identical to the pyogenic granuloma and often occurs on the gingivae at about the third month of pregnancy. The lesion gradually increases in size, but after delivery it may regress. If removal is attempted during pregnancy it may recur.

Treatment

Pyogenic granulomata are removed surgically, but this can be difficult, because there is no clear anatomical limit to the lesion. If on the gingivae, the base of the lesion needs to be thoroughly curetted and any contributory factors (such as the sharp edge of a tooth) removed.

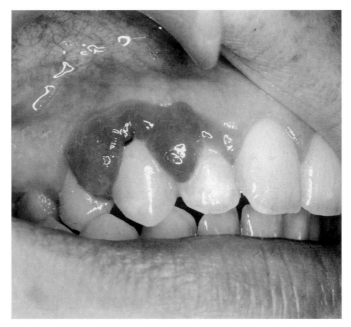

Fig. 6.5 Pregnancy tumour.

Peripheral giant cell granuloma (Fig. 6.6)

Aetiology

Confusingly named, this lesion is thought to be a response to local chronic irritation, although a precise cause is often not obvious.

Appearance

The lesion occurs on the gingivae, normally anterior to the molars, and its appearance may be similar to the fibrous epulis and the pyogenic granuloma. It is attached to deeper tissues such as periosteum or periodontal ligament, whereas the other lesions are attached to the surface gingivae. The surface of the lesion is often dusky red, because of its vascularity, and may often appear ulcerated.

Histology

The microscopic appearance is a non-encapsulated vascular lesion of spindle cells with an abundance of multinucleated giant cells. There may be spicules of newly formed bone or osteoid tissue lying within an extensive network of blood vessels.

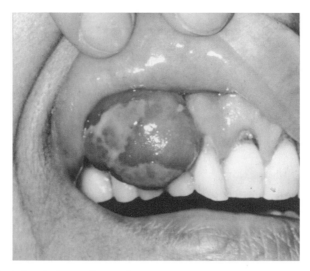

Fig. 6.6   Peripheral giant cell granuloma.

Treatment

Surgical excision, combined with the removal of the base of the granuloma, is the only satisfactory way of dealing with the lesion. As the lesion is non-encapsulated, a margin of normal tissue is also excised to prevent recurrence.

Denture granuloma (fibroma, hypertrophy, hyperplasia) (Fig. 6.7(a) and (b) (*see also* Chapter 12)

Aetiology

Poorly fitting dentures may be the cause of an inflammatory reactive hyperplasia when the periphery of the denture extends too deeply into the sulcus.

Clinical appearance

There is an elongated firm mass of rolled mucosa, typically found in the buccal sulcus, with the indentation of the flange of the denture present in its midst. The area may be painful, and the granuloma is flattened against the adjacent ridge due to the pressure from the denture. The lesion grows slowly and may show signs of ulceration on its surface.

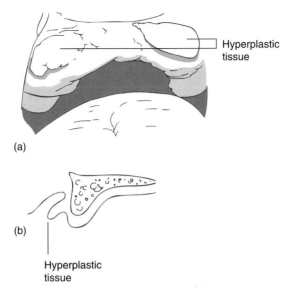

Fig. 6.7(a) and (b)   Denture granuloma of upper labial sulcus caused by an ill fitting denture.

Treatment

Initially, the denture should either not be worn, or its periphery cut back to prevent further trauma to the soft tissue. Following this measure there will often be considerable regression of the granuloma, and after a suitable interval, any remaining hyperplastic tissue can be excised. Dentures may have to be altered or remade to prevent the problem recurring.

Ulcers

The most common benign lesion found in the mouth is the ulcer, and an ulcer is produced when there is a break in the continuity of the oral epithelium. The oral epithelium is constantly subject to trauma, by the potentially damaging actions of chewing and swallowing hot or hard foods. It is surprising therefore that oral ulceration is not more common than it is.

Oral ulceration may be:

■ Confined to the mouth
■ Associated with skin lesions
■ Manifestations of systemic disease

A full description of all the conditions associated with oral ulceration would be inappropriate here, and only the commoner ulcers, confined to the mouth, will be considered. Most ulcers are painful and may interfere with chewing, swallowing or even speech.

Traumatic ulcers **(Fig. 6.8)**
These ulcers are single, ragged and painful. A history and examination will reveal the aetiology, and removal of the cause will result in a resolution of the ulcer. Common causes are toothbrush trauma, cheek biting, broken teeth and ill-fitting dentures.

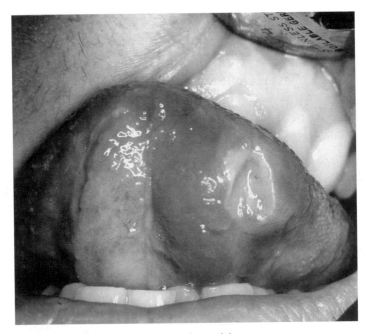

Fig. 6.8   Traumatic ulcer on the under surface of the tongue.

Primary herpetic gingivostomatitis
The oral mucosa is affected in the primary attack of the herpes simplex virus. The condition occurs in childhood, but can be seen in adults as well. The patient is febrile, and a crop of vesicles appears in any part of the mouth. These soon break down to form small ulcers, which may coalesce to produce a large ulcerated lesion. There is usually a gingivitis as well. The condition resolves in a week or so and palliative treatment with a high intake of fluids is all that is necessary. Recurrence of the condition can take the form of cold sores.

Recurrent oral ulceration

Minor aphthous ulcers (Fig. 6.9)

These affect women more than men, and frequently occur between 10 and 20 years of age. They may involve any area of the mouth, but commonly appear inside the lips and cheeks. After an initial burning or itching sensation, a crop of four or five small (4 to 6 mm) shallow ulcers, with a yellow floor and red margin, appears, typically inside the lips and cheeks or under the tongue. Healing takes between a week and 10 days, however in some patients the ulcers recur at regular intervals.

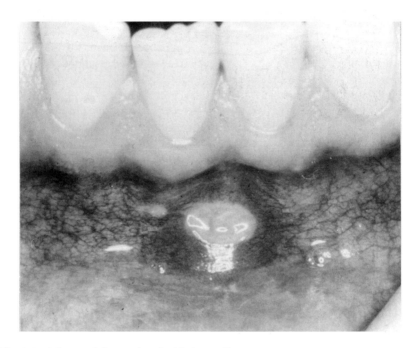

Fig. 6.9 Minor aphthous ulcer inside lower lip.

Major aphthous ulcers

These are a less common but more severe form of the minor variety. They tend to occur singly, are larger (1 to 5 cm) and take much longer to heal, often with scarring. These lesions can occur on the tongue and palate as well as the lips and cheeks.

Herpetiform ulcers

These appear as a crop of numerous shallow minute (2 to 3 mm) ulcers, which may coalesce to form a larger ulcer. They may look similar to the ulcers in acute herpetic gingivostomatitis, but a viral aetiology has not been established.

Treatment

As the aetiology of these ulcers has not been established, treatment is not curative. Topical steroid therapy using lozenges, mouthwash or spray is the mainstay of treatment and will reduce the timespan and severity of these lesions. Occasionally an underlying haematological abnormality may be found (iron, folate or B_{12} deficiency).

White patches and leukoplakia

Many conditions produce oral white patches and some of the terms used are not particularly helpful. Most are of no great significance, but the clinical appearance can be deceptive, and if any doubt exists, biopsy must always be considered to exclude pre-malignant change. In general terms, white patches occur when the surface layers of the mucous membrane are thickened (hyperkeratosis), usually in response to a specific stimulus or condition.

Traumatic lesions

- **Frictional keratosis:** white patches caused by local irritation, from dentures, sharp teeth or cheek biting, are common. White patches from cheek biting appear on the buccal mucosa, usually in the line of the occlusal plane.
- **Thermal and chemical injury:** an aspirin tablet placed adjacent to a tooth to control toothache will produce a chemical burn presenting initially as a white patch.
- **Smokers' keratosis** (Fig. 6.10): can be considered to be a result of thermal and chemical irritation. There is a whitish area in the palate with multiple red pinpoints representing the inflamed orifices of the minor salivary glands.
- **Alcoholic white patches:** can occur anywhere in the mouth.
- **Poor oral hygiene:** produces white patches around the teeth and on the gingivae.

Lichen planus

Oral lichen planus is a common, often symptomless, condition producing white patches. It usually affects the buccal mucosa or tongue. The clinical appearance varies from a fine, lacy pattern to thick white patches. There may also be red erosive areas. Malignant change can occasionally occur and biopsy of suspicious areas must be carried out.

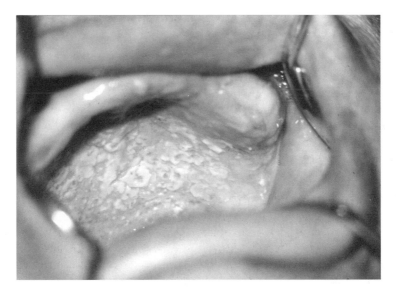

Fig. 6.10 Smokers' keratosis of palate.

Candidal infection

There are several clinical pictures in this condition, but acute pseudo-membranous candidosis (thrush) produces white patches in the cheek and palate which can be easily wiped off leaving a raw mucosal surface underneath. Chronic hyperplastic candidosis (candidal leukoplakia) produce white patches that do not wipe away and characteristically occur inside the corners of the mouth.

Leukoplakia

This is a term which should be reserved for a white patch which does not fit clinically or histologically into any of the other categories. It is a clinical term only, but tends to be used in connection with histological abnormality and malignant potential. Biopsy is essential to exclude pre-malignant change (dysplasia), especially in leukoplakia affecting the floor of the mouth and undersurface of the tongue. If treatment is necessary, laser vaporisation is a very useful technique for these lesions which are often extensive and superficial.

Hairy leukoplakia of the tongue raises the possibility of HIV infection.

White sponge naevus

This is a rare hereditary condition producing thick white patches throughout the mouth.

Haemangioma (Fig. 6.11)

A haemangioma is a vascular malformation, characterised by a proliferation of blood vessels, which may be present at birth or not develop
until old age. Several different types exist (for example capillary
haemangioma, cavernous haemangioma).

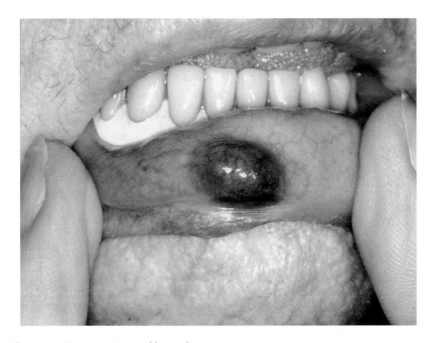

Fig. 6.11   Haemangioma of lower lip.

Clinical appearance

In the mouth, a haemangioma may appear as a localised raised lesion and
may be on the lips, tongue, buccal mucosa or palate. It is obviously blood-
filled and compressible.

Rare, but potentially dangerous haemangiomatous conditions are:

- **Sturge-Weber syndrome:** present at birth, this condition involves
  haemangiomas of the mouth and upper face with intracranial exten-
  sions of the lesions.
- **Hereditary haemorrhagic telangectasia** is a condition characterised
  by the appearance in adult life of multiple small vascular lesions in the
  oral cavity, nasal cavity and skin.
- **Bony haemangioma** can be life threatening.

Treatment

This is not always necessary, but the majority of oral lesions respond to the cryoprobe. Lasers may also be used. Very extensive lesions are treated by embolisation, with or without surgery.

Frenectomy

A frenum is a band of mucosa and fibrous tissue passing from the lips, cheeks or tongue to the alveolar ridge. These are normal structures usually obvious in the midline between the upper lip and ridge, and also between the undersurface of the tongue and lower jaw. If the upper labial frenum is hyperplastic it may produce separation of the upper incisors or interfere with the fit of an upper denture. A hyperplastic lingual frenum may restrict the movement of the tongue ('tongue tie').

Upper labial frenectomy involves the removal of a small amount of soft tissue from between the upper central incisors and also the band of mucosa crossing the sulcus between the alveolar ridge and lip (Fig. 6.12).

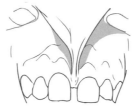

Fig. 6.12   Hyperplastic upper labial frenum.

Lingual frenectomy involves division of the tight band of tissue tethering the tongue to the lower jaw (Fig. 6.13). No tissue is removed. A Z-plasty may be used for repair but is generally not necessary. Care needs to be taken to avoid damage to the submandibular ducts and blood vessels in the floor of the mouth at the base of the frenum.

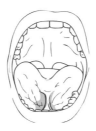

Fig. 6.13   Tongue tie.

Management techniques

Biopsy (*see also* Chapter 11, Part I)

- Biopsy involves the removal of a representative sample of tissue for histological examination, as an aid to or confirmation of the clinical diagnosis.
- Wherever possible, some normal tissue should be included in the specimen.
- Incisional biopsy involves removal of only part of the lesion, usually a sample from the edge (Fig. 6.14). A deep, narrow biopsy is generally preferable to a broad, shallow one.
- Excisional biopsy attempts to remove the whole lesion, and is often the treatment of choice for small, benign soft tissue lesions (Fig. 6.15). The wound can usually be closed primarily without difficulty.
- Specimens are placed immediately in formol saline (formalin), with markers (e.g. a suture) for orientation if necessary.
- An accurate record and diagram of the site and type of biopsy should be made.

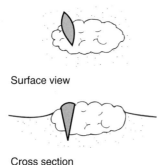

Surface view

Cross section

Fig. 6.14(a) and (b)   Incisional biopsy.

Cryosurgery

This involves the use of extreme cold in treatment, cell death occurring below –20°C. Commonly used systems employ nitrous oxide and probes of various shapes and sizes to suit the lesion being treated. For most lesions two freeze–thaw cycles are used.

There are no immediate visible effects, but over 24 hours swelling and discoloration occur, followed by formation of a yellowish slough after 2 days. Complete healing in the mouth can take up to 3 weeks, but is with minimal or no scarring.

It is possible to use cryosurgery for a wide range of oral and skin

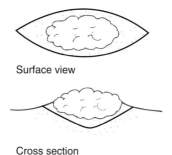

Surface view

Cross section

Fig. 6.15(a) and (b) Excisional biopsy.

lesions, but haemangiomas respond very satisfactorily. Mucous cysts can also be treated successfully. Polyps, papillomas and granulomas may also be treated, although surgical excision is generally the treatment of choice. It must be remembered that no specimen for histological examination is produced during cryotherapy, although biopsy can be carried out before treatment.

Treatment is usually carried out on an out-patient basis and an example is given of cryosurgery for a haemangioma of the lip.

Pre-operative preparation of the patient

Patient information and informed consent with special reference to swelling of the lip and slough formation, its effect on speech and feeding, and the time scale involved (Information leaflet No 9).

Procedure

Equipment/instruments required

- Cryosurgical machine and probes (Fig. 6.17). The nitrous oxide supply should be checked and turned on, and a suitable probe connected and tested.
- K-Y gel may be used to increase thermal conductivity although this is not usually necessary in the mouth.
- Suitable retractors. Dental mirrors are usually adequate.
- Suitable drapes.

Anaesthesia

Local anaesthesia may be given although for many oral lesions no anaesthetic is necessary.

PATIENT INFORMATION LEAFLET No 9

ORAL and MAXILLOFACIAL SURGERY DEPARTMENT

CRYOTHERAPY

- Cryotherapy is the treatment of lesions by freezing using a small probe.
- The lesion is usually frozen for approximately 2 minutes followed by a break of about one minute after which the lesion is again frozen for 2 minutes.
- No local anaesthetic injection is necessary although there may be a slight twinge as freezing starts, and an aching sensation as the tissues thaw.
- No immediate effects are noticeable, but over the first 24 hours there will be some swelling, discoloration and discomfort. After 2 or 3 days the area may become 'sloughy'.
- Treatment of a lesion on the lips or tongue may temporarily affect speech and feeding.
- Painkillers e.g. paracetamol are usually necessary for several days, and a mouthwash should be used if the treated area is inside the mouth.
- Healing takes up to 2 weeks.
- A review appointment will be given.
- Further freezing is sometimes necessary.
- If you have any problems after treatment please ring . . . . for advice.

Position

Standard in dental chair.

Operative procedure

- The probe is applied to the lesion and sticks to the tissues as soon as freezing starts. Care must be taken to retract and protect adjacent soft tissue.
- A visible iceball will form in the tissues at the tip of the probe (Fig. 6.16). The timing and number of freeze–thaw cycles will vary

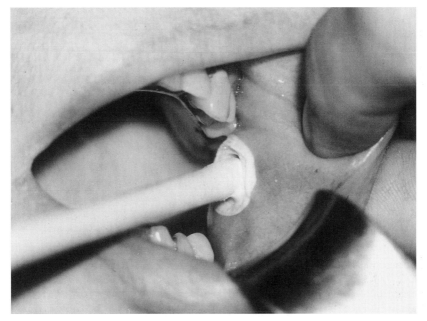

Fig. 6.16 Cryoprobe applied to lesion.

according to the size and nature of the lesion being treated, but for a small haemangioma, two freeze–thaw cycles of 2 minutes each are adequate.
■ Thawing should take place before any attempt is made to remove the probe.

Post-operative care and follow-up

■ Written post-operative instructions
■ Analgesia and antiseptic mouthwash
■ Follow-up appointment

Laser surgery

Lasers will be considered in this section, although their use is not confined to the treatment of benign soft tissue lesions. Several types of laser (Light Amplification of Stimulated Emission of Radiation) systems exist, including those for dermatological surgery. Within the specialty, however, the CO_2 and Nd:YAG are the main systems in use. YAG lasers penetrate more deeply and can produce more damage in the surrounding normal tissue than CO_2 lasers, which are ideal for surface vaporisation of

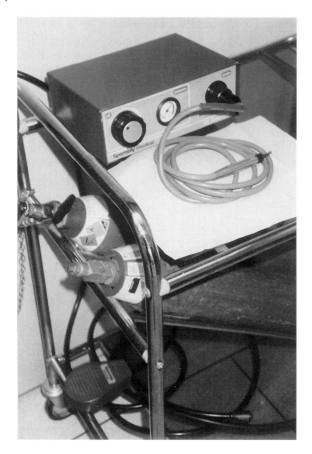

Fig. 6.17   Cryosurgical machine and probe.

superficial lesions. Both systems produce a relatively bloodless field by coagulating and sealing blood vessels as cutting proceeds. Laser wounds show less inflammation than other wounds and this can mean less pain, swelling and scar formation, but a slightly slower rate of healing.

Safety aspects

- Local protocols will exist following national guidelines (a legal requirement).
- **Patients:** penetration of the endotracheal tube by the laser beam and ignition of the anaesthetic gases is the most serious risk. Armoured tubes may be used or metal foil and saline soaked gauze packs used to protect normal tubes. Eyes are protected with saline soaked pads and plastic eye shields.
- **Staff:** all involved must be appropriately trained. Special goggles are

mandatory for the YAG laser, but normal spectacles or simple goggles are adequate for the CO_2 laser. Warning signs must be displayed at operating theatre entrances. Very highly polished instruments or retractors must not be used and the laser kept on standby mode at all times when not actually being used.

Summary

- A wide range of benign soft tissue lesions is encountered in the mouth.
- Most requiring surgery are treated on an out-patient basis under local anaesthetic.
- Biopsy is often a crucial procedure for diagnosis.
- Patients are frequently extremely anxious about the possibility of malignancy.

7

Surgery for Jaw Deformity

P. Cove

Jaw deformity is an abnormality of growth and development and can range from a minor variation to severe disproportion or asymmetry. It usually develops during childhood and may become more noticeable during puberty. Some deformities may be present at birth, for example cleft lip and palate.

Jaw deformity

Dentofacial deformity may produce a number of problems for the patient which broadly fall into two categories. Functional problems include difficulty with mastication and speech and poor dental health due to malocclusion. Aesthetic problems may be severe enough to interfere significantly with the patient's social or psychological well-being. Orthognathic surgery aims to correct jaw deformity or disproportion using a range of surgical procedures selected on an individual basis for each patient. Treatment may extend for up to two years and frequently involves pre- and post-operative orthodontics. Management is essentially a team effort with contributions from experienced nurses in the outpatient department, the ward and operating theatre, anaesthetists and maxillofacial technicians, as well as the orthodontist and surgeon.

Classification

- Maxillary protrusion
- Maxillary retrusion
- Mandibular protrusion
- Mandibular retrusion
- Asymmetry of mandible
- Facial asymmetry

Management

Indications for surgery

- To improve jaw function
- To improve facial harmony
- To assist speech

Treatment planning

Patients are seen in joint clinics by surgeons and orthodontists and a treatment plan agreed which typically includes pre-operative orthodontics, surgery and post-operative orthodontics. Surgery does not normally take place until facial growth is complete in the mid to late teens, and treatment may extend over a period of 2 years.

Assessment of the patients includes the following:

- Patient motivation. The surgeon will wish to find out what the patient sees as the problems, what is expected from treatment and whether the patient is sufficiently motivated to undertake the prolonged orthodontic treatment and the surgery. The assessment involves at least some psychological evaluation.

- Evaluation of the patient's medical status.
- Preparation of study casts in plaster of the teeth and jaws.
- Radiographs of the jaws and facial bones. Tracings of the lateral skull radiographs are prepared, usually by computer.
- Computed tomographic (CT) scanning and sometimes bone scans may be required, for example in cases of asymmetry.
- Many patients are at school and it is essential to keep parents fully informed at all times so that they are in the best position to guide and advise their children. For children and students surgery is often planned around their academic and family commitments.
- Maxillofacial laboratory. Maxillofacial technicians play an important part in the pre-operative planning and preparation of patients undergoing surgery for jaw deformity. The plaster casts of the teeth and jaws are specially prepared so that the dental occlusion following surgery can be predicted. These predictions are combined with the computer tracings of the radiographs so that the final surgical plan can be decided. At this stage the occlusal wafers (templates), which are used during surgery, are constructed.

Pre-operative preparation of patient

- Pre-admission clinics. Patients usually attend the pre-admission clinic about 4 weeks before surgery. Agreed protocols are used by the nurses working on these clinics and ideally the consultant in charge of the patient carries out a full review of the patient at the same time. Most patients are admitted to the ward on the day prior to surgery, but with the above preparation many can be admitted on the day of surgery.
- Patient information (*see* Information leaflet No 10). The surgical plan will have been explained several times by the time the patient has been admitted. The main points are again discussed and any questions answered.
- Consent with special reference to swelling, nerve damage and the possibility of the jaws being fixed together.
- Standard checklist for general anaesthetic.
- All clinical photographs, radiographs, study casts and splints or occlusal wafers must be available.
- Dietitian – usually sees patient and relatives prior to surgery.
- The hygienist may see the patient pre-operatively.

PATIENT INFORMATION LEAFLET No 10

ORTHOGNATHIC SURGERY

Orthognathic surgery is carried out to improve the alignment of the jaws.

Why do I need jaw surgery combined with orthodontics?

The objectives of orthodontics, or 'straightening' of your teeth, are sometimes limited by the position of the jaws in which the teeth lie. Correction of one or both jaws, by surgery, allows the teeth to be positioned better when this cannot be done by orthodontics alone. This also improves the function of the teeth and jaws as a chewing system and the general facial appearance.

   At the joint Orthodontic/Maxillofacial Surgery clinics, the option of this combined approach to achieve the best possible result will be discussed with you. Both techniques must be planned together and choosing this treatment requires a considerable commitment.

SEQUENCE OF PLANNING AND TREATMENT

1. Assessment, Planning and Discussion
   The Orthodontists and Maxillofacial Surgeons will discuss your concerns and the long-term aim of your treatment.

2. Pre-surgical Orthodontics (The Orthodontic Team)
   Fixed braces will move your teeth in each arch into better positions in preparation for surgery to one or both jaws. The teeth will then fit and function better. This stage usually takes between one and two years.

3. Orthognathic Surgery (The Surgical Team)
   You will be admitted to the ward the day before the operation.

▶

PATIENT INFORMATION LEAFLET No 10 *continued*

Jaw surgery is carried out while you are asleep under a general anaesthetic. You can expect to spend from 3 to 7 days in hospital, where you will recover after the operation with expert supervision and then be allowed home. You would be wise to arrange a month off work or school/college, during which time you will be reviewed weekly to monitor and assess your progress, extending to monthly reviews after this period.

All the surgery is performed within the mouth, cuts made along the gum allow the bones of the jaw to be moved into the correct position. They are fixed with small metal plates and screws which usually remain in the bone. They may sometimes need to be removed at a later date if causing a mild problem. The correct jaw position is achieved using a thin clear plastic splint or 'wafer', which usually remains secured to the lower teeth for some weeks. Dissolving stitches neatly close the gum. When you wake from your anaesthetic you can open your mouth, but gentle elastic bands are placed the next day using the braces on the upper and lower teeth to guide your teeth into the bite-wafer. These elastics are replaced with fresh ones, by us initially, and by you later at home. Occasionally, it may be necessary to wire the jaws together after the operation for a short period.

As with any operation, you can expect some discomfort and swelling. This will start during the first two days, beginning to settle over the next week or two. Painkillers are given to control any discomfort and you will have some to take home.

Great care is taken to protect the nerves of feeling that run through the jaws at the time of surgery, but you may experience areas of facial numbness immediately post-operatively. If the upper jaw is moved, the numb feeling is limited to the cheeks and upper lip; if the lower jaw is moved, it is limited to the lower lip and chin, and possibly the tongue. This reduced sensation or 'paraesthesia' will return to normal over the ensuing weeks or months. Very rarely, an area of permanently dulled or altered sensation remains. Appearance and movement of the face are not affected, as the nerves to the facial muscles are not involved in the area of operation.

Specialist assistance is provided by:

The Dental Hygienist or Dental Health Educator to help you keep your mouth and braces clean.

▶

PATIENT INFORMATION LEAFLET No 10 *continued*

The Dietitian will advise on nutritious soft and liquid diets essential for good healing and recovery. You will need a blender at home for frequent, smaller meals, as your intake will be limited initially.

You should be up and about within a day or two and back to your normal routine within a month and will appreciate the improvement in your face as the swelling resolves completely. The jaw bones are completely healed after 2 to 3 months.

4. *Post-surgical Orthodontics (The Orthodontic Team)*
A period of further orthodontic treatment is usually required to fine-tune tooth alignment and obtain the best fit of the upper and lower teeth in the new position of the jaws. This may take 3 to 12 months, after which the fixed braces are removed. A period of settling of the teeth takes place and retainers are needed to control unwanted tooth movement. A removable type of retainer is used in the upper jaw and can be removed for cleaning. In the lower, a discreet fixed retainer glued behind the lower front teeth may be used for up to a year.

This leaflet is aimed as an introduction. If you have any further questions please raise these at your next appointment. Please feel free to bring a written list.

Surgery to reduce the size of the lower jaw

Surgery to advance the lower jaw and chin

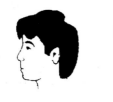
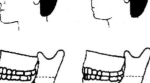
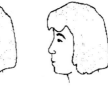
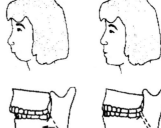

Operating theatre procedure

Instruments required

- Intra-oral set (*see* Fig. 4.5)
- Osteotomy set (*see* Fig. 4.9)
- Wiring set (*see* Fig. 4.11)
- Plating system (*see* Fig. 4.12)
- Drill/saw system (*see* Figs 4.13 and 4.14)
- Local anaesthetic for infiltration

Anaesthesia

Naso-tracheal intubation. Hypotensive anaesthesia may be required.

Position

Standard for intra-oral procedure.

Preparation of operative site

- Standard peri-oral preparation
- Standard head towel and drapes

Procedures on the maxilla

Osteotomies may be at the Le Fort I, II and III levels (Fig. 7.1). This classification was named after Rene Le Fort – a surgeon who carried out research on cadavers in Paris (published in 1901) – and was originally applied to fractures of the maxilla.

Osteotomies at the Le Fort II and III levels are carried out less commonly and only the Le Fort I osteotomy is described. The maxilla may be moved in any direction to correct the particular discrepancy being treated.

Le Fort 1 maxillary osteotomy

Operative procedure

- The sulcus area is infiltrated with local anaesthetic, e.g. 2% lignocaine with 1 in 200 000 adrenaline.
- An incision is made (Fig. 7.2) in the sulcus and the periosteum reflected to expose the nasal aperture and lateral surfaces of the

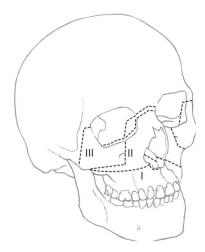

Fig. 7.1   The Le Fort osteotomy lines in the upper facial skeleton.

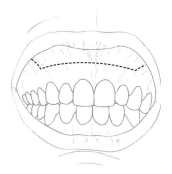

Fig. 7.2   Mucosal incision for Le Fort maxillary osteotomy.

maxilla. The nasal mucoperiosteum is also reflected from the floor of the nose and the base of the nasal septum.

- Bone cuts are carried out using a fine reciprocating saw (Fig. 7.3). The nasal septum is separated from the palate with a septal chisel and a fine osteotome is used to cut the lateral nasal walls. Finally the maxilla is separated from the pterygoid bones with a curved osteotome.
- The maxilla is fractured downwards and any sharp edges removed with bone rongeurs and/or burs (Fig. 7.4).
- The maxilla is mobilised and moved to the new planned position and temporarily fixed to the mandible with intermaxillary tie wires or elastics (IMF), and an occlusal wafer (template) between the teeth to confirm the accuracy of the position.
- The maxilla is fixed with bone plates (Fig. 7.5), the IMF is released and the new dental occlusion checked.

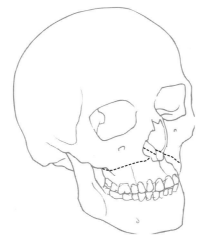

Fig. 7.3 Bone cuts for Le Fort maxillary osteotomy.

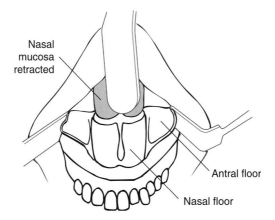

Fig. 7.4 Maxilla downfractured showing floor of nose and maxillary antra.

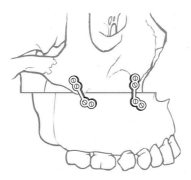

Fig. 7.5 Maxilla fixed in new position with bone plates.

■ The incision is closed with resorbable sutures.
■ Any throat packing is removed and the pharynx cleared by suction and the lips lubricated with petroleum jelly.

Post-operative care

■ **Airway:** as with all jaw surgery, protection of the airway is the first priority. Monitoring is carried in the recovery area and continues when the patient returns to the ward. If patients have their jaws wired together it is mandatory that wire cutting equipment accompanies the patient at all times in the initial recovery period. Patients whose jaws are wired together are usually kept in the high dependency unit for the first 24 hours.
■ **Haemorrhage:** the second priority relates to haemorrhage, which may threaten the airway. Packing may be required for epistaxis. Frequent monitoring is required in these cases.
■ **Swelling:** moderate facial oedema is normal after these procedures. It can be reduced by the administration of dexamethazone during the operation and for 24 to 48 hours post-operatively. Ice packs and elevation of the head of the bed also help.
■ **Pain control:** suitable analgesia, ideally in a dispersible form, is pre-scribed and anti-inflammatory drugs are given. As well as their analgesic effect, anti-inflammatory agents will also reduce swelling.
■ **Prevention of infection:** antibiotic prophylaxis is normally given for this type of surgery.
■ **Oral hygiene:** good oral hygiene is important in the prevention of infection, and chlorhexidine mouth baths are commenced on the first post-operative day.
■ **Diet:** oral function is initially compromised, but quickly returns to normal. A suitable regime is:

1st 12 hours	IV fluids
12 to 24 hours	oral fluids
24 hours onwards	soft diet

■ **Dental occlusion** is monitored and patients often find that gentle elastic traction, on hooks or brackets attached to the teeth, will help support the jaw in its new position. Minor discrepancies in the occlusion may also be corrected in this way.

Complications

■ **Nerve damage** causing paraesthesia (altered sensation) or anaesthesia occurs commonly after orthognathic surgery. Fortunately nerve function largely recovers but all patients have to be warned of the possibility before surgery is undertaken. Care must be taken to remind patients of the danger of burning their mouths or faces during the post-operative phase.

- **Infection:** bony infection is rare, but non-union at an osteotomy site may occur. Bone plates or screws may need to be removed because of infection.
- **Relapse:** failure to maintain the new planned position of the jaw may be caused by technical errors during fixation. In the longer term the altered forces exerted by the lips and tongue on the teeth in their new position may cause slight tooth movement.

Follow-up

This is frequent at first, for example weekly, and is gradually reduced. The patient returns to the care of the orthodontist for management of the occlusion including the final orthodontic phase. The patients continue to be reviewed at combined clinics by surgeons and orthodontists for a number of years.

Procedures on the mandible

Osteotomies may be carried out on the angle and ascending ramus of the mandible (sagittal split and vertical subsigmoid osteotomies) and on the body of the mandible. There are now few indications for body osteotomy. The mandible may be advanced, set back or rotated depending on the discrepancy being treated.

Sagittal split osteotomy

Operative procedure

- The operative sites are infiltrated with lignocaine with 1 in 200 000 adrenaline, and the angle and part of the ascending ramus is exposed via an incision in the third molar region.
- The periosteum is widely reflected from the areas of the bony cuts.
- Using burs or saws the inner cortical plate of the ascending ramus of the jaw is cut horizontally above the level of the lingula and the outer plate is cut vertically level with the second molar. The two cuts are now joined with a third cut down the anterior border of the angle of the jaw. The same procedure is now carried out on the other side (Fig. 7.6).
- The mandibular rami are split on each side using a range of osteotomes and bone spreading instruments, taking great care to preserve the neurovascular bundle running within the mandible (Fig. 7.7).

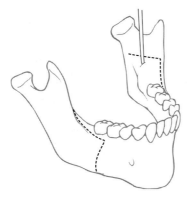

Fig. 7.6   Bony cuts for sagittal split osteotomy. The cuts are only in the outer cortex of the bone.

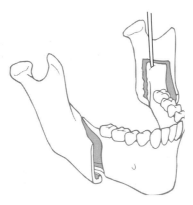

Fig. 7.7   Bony splits completed.

- The body of the mandible is repositioned and temporarily fixed to the maxilla with intermaxillary tie wires or elastics (IMF) and an occlusal wafer (template) between the teeth to confirm the accuracy of the position.
- The body of the mandible is fixed in its new position with bone plates or screws, the IMF released and the occlusion checked (Fig. 7.8).
- Small vacuum drains may be placed and the wounds closed with resorbable sutures.
- Any throat packing is removed and the mouth and pharynx cleared by suction and the lips lubricated with petroleum jelly.

Post-operative care, complications and follow-up

These are as previously described and similar to a maxillary osteotomy.

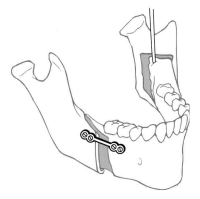

Fig. 7.8 Mandible fixed in new position with bone plates.

Vertical subsigmoid osteotomy

This osteotomy is carried out on the posterior part of the angle and ascending ramus of the mandible. An intra-oral approach using an angled saw is usual, although an extra-oral approach is possible (Fig. 7.9(a) and (b)).

Bimaxillary procedures

Surgery on one jaw may be insufficient to correct the deformity and osteotomies on both upper and lower jaws (bimaxillary) are required.

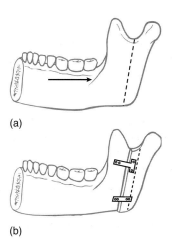

(a)

(b)

Fig. 7.9 Vertical subsigmoid osteotomy (a) Mandibular cut; (b) overlap and fixation.

Operative procedure

■ The mandibular bone cuts are made first but the ramus splitting is deferred until the maxillary osteotomy has been completed and the maxilla fixed in its new position.
■ The mandibular rami are then split and the mandible is repositioned and fixed as before.
■ The wounds in both jaws are then closed.

Note: two occlusal wafers are required, intermediate and final.

Segmental procedures

The dentoalveolar sections of either jaw can be mobilised and repositioned. The segments are stabilised using the remaining (stable) part of the jaw and a combination of bone plates and dental splinting.

The maxilla

The anterior maxilla may be repositioned, usually to correct maxillary protrusion (Fig 7.10). A pre-molar tooth is extracted on each side and access to the palatal bone is made by tunnelling under the muco-periosteum. Bone is removed with burs to allow the segment to be repositioned and fixation can be carried out using arch bars, plates or an acrylic plate.

The posterior dentoalveolar segment may be intruded to correct anterior open bite defects. Fixation is similar to that used for anterior segmental procedures (Fig. 7.11).

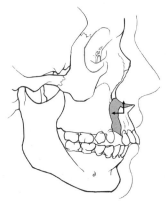

Fig. 7.10   Anterior maxillary osteotomy to correct maxillary protrusion.

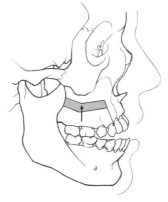

Fig. 7.11 Posterior maxillary osteotomy to correct anterior open bite.

The mandible

The anterior mandible is usually repositioned inferiorly and posteriorly to correct over eruption and protrusion of the lower incisor segment. Care is needed to avoid damaging the mental nerves (Fig. 7.12).

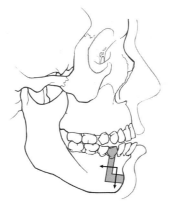

Fig. 7.12 Anterior mandibular osteotomy to correct protrusion of lower incisor teeth.

Genioplasty

These operations are designed to augment or reduce the chin prominence (Fig. 7.13(a) and (b)), and may be part of a treatment plan which includes surgery to the rest of the lower jaw or both jaws. Control of the overlying soft tissues is difficult to achieve but it is best done by avoiding stripping all the soft tissues from the chin. Post-operatively a pressure dressing is applied to the chin.

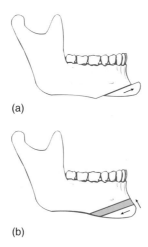

(a)

(b)

Fig. 7.13   (a) Augmentation genioplasty; (b) reduction genioplasty.

Distraction osteogenesis

Originally described by a Russian surgeon, Ilizarov, this technique uses slow distraction at an osteotomy site to induce new bone formation. Its application is mainly in congenital conditions producing severe maxillofacial skeletal deficiency, notably hemifacial microsomia. This syndrome manifests as a deficiency of bone and soft tissue in the region of the posterior mandible and ear.

The mandible

The mandible is exposed either intra-orally or externally and most of the outer cortical plate of bone at the osteotomy site is cut with a bur. An expansion device is fitted to both sides of the cut and the osteotomy is completed (Fig. 7.14). The two halves of the expansion device are connected by a screw system and the wounds are closed.

Approximately one week after surgery the screw is turned so that the bone is lengthened by a small amount each day until the required length is achieved (Fig. 7.15). After a further period the appliance can be removed.

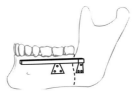

Fig. 7.14   Distraction osteogenesis. Distractor fitted across osteotomy.

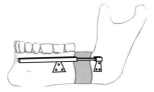

Fig. 7.15 Mandible lengthened by bony distraction.

This technique can be used for increasing the length or height of the jaw. Intra-oral appliances are likely to be more acceptable to the patient, but external distractors may give better control of bone movement.

The maxilla

The approach to the maxilla is similar to that employed for maxillary osteotomies. Following the osteotomy cuts, forward traction is applied to the maxilla using a cranial or facial frame to advance the upper jaw into the correct position.

Summary

The correction of jaw deformity involves prolonged treatment and major elective surgery. The patient's expectations of the functional and aesthetic improvements to be gained will usually be high and the nurses' contribution to pre-operative information and counselling form an important part of the overall treatment.

The complicated nature of the surgery makes the nurses' role in the operating theatre vital for the successful execution of orthognathic surgery. In the immediate post-operative period patients require close monitoring, especially of the airway, and later, sympathetic support during what for many patients is a difficult period.

8

Salivary Glands

C. Yates

This chapter gives a brief outline of the structure and function of the salivary glands. Their disorders are described with emphasis on those requiring surgical management.

Structure of the salivary glands

The major salivary glands comprise three large paired glands (Fig. 8.1):

■ Parotid
■ Submandibular
■ Sublingual

Together these glands secrete approximately 1500 ml of saliva daily.

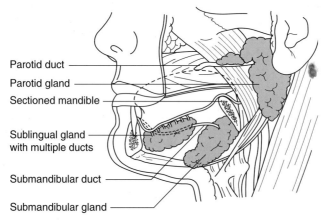

Parotid duct
Parotid gland
Sectioned mandible

Sublingual gland
with multiple ducts

Submandibular duct

Submandibular gland

Fig. 8.1   The major salivary glands.

The parotid gland is irregularly wedge shaped and lies in the space between the posterior border of the ramus of the mandible and the sternomastoid muscle below the external auditory meatus. Anteriorly the gland overlaps the masseter muscle and from this part of the gland the parotid duct runs forward to open into the mouth opposite the upper second molar tooth. Important structures within the gland are the external carotid artery and the facial nerve.

The submandibular gland is also irregularly shaped, projecting beneath the lower border of the mandible but extending above, medial to the mandible almost reaching the mouth in the molar region. The submandibular duct runs forward along the floor of the mouth for about 5 cm to open on a papilla at the side of the frenulum of the tongue close to the midline. The facial artery and the lingual and hypoglossal nerves are closely related to the submandibular gland.

The sublingual gland lies in the floor of the mouth just beneath the mucosa, producing a ridge – the sublingual fold. The gland is elongated and reaches from the midline curving around the inner aspect of the mandible to reach the submandibular gland behind. Between 10 and 20 sublingual ducts open into the mouth along the sublingual fold. Closely related to the gland are the submandibular duct and the lingual nerve.

The minor salivary glands are mucus secreting and situated submucosally in the lips, cheeks, hard and soft palates and tongue. There are between 200 and 300 minor salivary glands.

Disorders of the salivary glands

Obstruction

Obstruction of the minor salivary glands most commonly occurs in the lower lip, usually in connection with minor trauma. A mucous cyst results and treatment is by excision of the cyst together with the mucous gland in the base of the cyst.

The major salivary glands become obstructed by calculi in the glands themselves or in their ducts. Obstruction of salivary flow will cause swelling of the affected gland, typically at mealtimes.

Stones in the ducts may be removed and the gland return to normal function. Stones within the glands themselves, if producing symptoms, will usually necessitate removal of the gland, although this may not be so for the parotid gland. Minor obstructive episodes may be managed conservatively.

Infection

Infection may be viral (mumps) or bacterial. Bacterial infection often arises in association with obstruction, or in debilitated patients when salivary flow is decreased. Management may be conservative, using antibiotics although drainage will be necessary if there is abscess formation.

Tumours

Benign and malignant tumours occur in both minor and major salivary glands. The commonest benign tumour is the pleomorphic adenoma and this can occur at any site, but most commonly in the parotid gland and the minor salivary glands of the hard and soft palates.

A range of malignant tumours occur, chiefly adenoidcystic carcinoma, mucoepidermoid carcinoma and adenocarcinoma.

Treatment of all tumours is principally surgical with additional radiotherapy for malignant lesions.

Autoimmune disease

Sjögrens syndrome is an association of dry eyes due to decreased lachrymal secretion, dry mouth due to decreased salivary secretion, and a connective tissue disorder, usually arthritis. Salivary gland enlargement and malignancy may occur in this condition.

Major salivary gland surgery

Parotidectomy

Indications

- Tumours or obstructive or inflammatory disease
- Surgery may involve only the superficial part of the gland, or both superficial and deep lobes (total parotidectomy)

Diagnosis and Investigations

- Swelling, pain
- Facial weakness indicates a malignant tumour
- CT, MRI or ultrasound scanning
- Sialography (radiographs taken following injection of radio-opaque dye into the gland via the duct)
- Fine needle aspiration biopsy (FNAB)

Aims

Removal of tumour or diseased gland without damage to the facial nerve (this may not be possible in malignant tumours).

Pre-operative preparation of the patient

- Patient information and informed consent. Special reference given to facial weakness following surgery, and the loss of skin sensation in certain areas.
- The hair is shaved from in front of the ear and neck/mastoid area if necessary.

Operating theatre procedure

Instruments required

- Extra-oral tissue set
- Skin marking pen and methylene blue for tattooing if required
- Local anaesthetic for skin infiltration
- Nerve stimulator

Anaesthesia

Endotracheal intubation with the tube placed in the opposite corner of the mouth. Hypotensive anaesthesia may be required.

Position

Standard, with head supported and turned away from the operating side.

Preparation of operative site

■ Skin preparation
■ Standard head towels to expose the whole of the side of the face and neck to the midline
■ Plug of cotton wool or foam in the ear

Operative procedure

The example given is for a standard superficial parotidectomy for a benign tumour in the tail of the gland.

■ The skin is marked and the incision line may be infiltrated with local anaesthetic (lignocaine with 1:200 000 adrenaline). Following incision (Fig. 8.2), a skin flap is raised to expose the whole of the parotid area including the tumour.
■ The next stage involves the identification of the main trunk of the facial nerve which arises deeply from between the bony external auditory canal and the mastoid process (Fig. 8.3). The area is approached by separating the posterior margin of the gland from the sternomastoid muscle, the mastoid process and the cartilaginous part of the external auditory meatus.

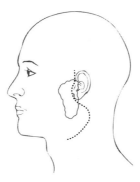

Fig. 8.2 Incision for parotidectomy.

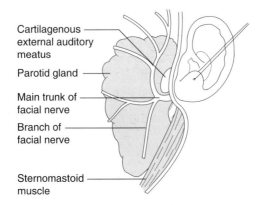

Cartilagenous external auditory meatus

Parotid gland

Main trunk of facial nerve

Branch of facial nerve

Sternomastoid muscle

Fig. 8.3   Identification of the facial nerve.

- Following identification of the nerve, dissection of the tumour can proceed with minimal risk to the nerve.
- After the tumour has been removed the wound is irrigated with saline, haemostasis is checked, a vacuum drain placed and the wound closed, usually in two layers.
- A pressure dressing may be used.

For tumours involving the deep portion of the gland, that is the gland beneath the plane of the facial nerve, the nerve is first identified as described, before dissection of the deep lobe takes place. The external carotid artery will need to be divided and occasionally a mandibular osteotomy is necessary for access.

Branches of the facial nerve which pass into a tumour are divided and may be repaired using a graft from the great auricular nerve which is dissected early in the procedure when the skin flap is raised.

Parotidectomy in continuity with a neck dissection may be carried out for malignant tumours.

Post-operative care

- If used, a pressure dressing is maintained for 48 hours
- Drains should be maintained until very little or no drainage is taking place
- Suture removal is between 5 and 7 days

Complications

Facial weakness
Dissection of the facial nerve will usually result in temporary facial weakness. Sacrifice of the nerve or its branches will produce permanent

loss of facial movement. Where repair of the facial nerve is impossible, or unsuccessful, fascial slings may be used to disguise facial asymmetry and a lateral tarsorrhaphy performed to protect the eye.

Skin sensation
The great auricular nerve is frequently divided during parotid surgery and will result in anaesthesia over the lower half of the ear. There will usually be some permanent deficit.

Salivary fistula
Remnants of normal glandular tissue may continue to secrete, and an accumulation of saliva in the wound or leakage at the incision line may result. Pressure dressing and combined drainage and aspiration may be necessary.

Frey syndrome
Inappropriate re-innervation of sweat glands in the skin of the parotid area by parasympathetic secretomotor nerve fibres from the parotid gland produces flushing or sweating of the skin with eating – gustatory sweating.

Operations on the parotid duct

- Calculi in the terminal parotid duct may be removed intra-orally through an incision over the duct.
- Calculi in the intra-glandular duct can be removed using a parotidectomy type approach, although it is not usually necessary to fully dissect the facial nerve.
- Strictures of the parotid duct (usually following infection or trauma) may be treated by dilatation using lachrymal probes. Stricture of the duct at its orifice may be relieved surgically by cutting down onto a probe placed in the terminal duct. To maintain the increased opening, the duct lining is sewn to the oral mucosa.

Removal of the submandibular gland

Indications

- Obstructive or inflammatory disease
- Tumours

Diagnosis and investigations

- Swelling, pain
- Plain X-rays for calculi

- CT, MRI or ultrasound scanning
- Sialography
- FNAB for suspected tumours

Aims

Removal of the gland without damage to associated nerves (this may not be possible with tumours).

Pre-operative preparation of the patient

Patient information and informed consent with special reference to facial weakness and tongue sensation.

Operating theatre procedure

Instruments required

- Extra-oral tissue set
- Lachrymal probes if intra-oral exploration of the duct is anticipated

Anaesthesia

Endotracheal with nasal intubation if intra-oral surgery is anticipated.

Position

Standard with head supported and turned away from the side of surgery. Neck slightly extended.

Preparation of operative site

- Standard skin preparation
- Standard head towels

Operative procedure

The example given is for removal of a submandibular gland for chronic obstruction or infection.

- The skin incision is marked and may be infiltrated with local anaesthetic (Fig. 8.4). Skin and subcutaneous fat, platysma muscle and deep fascia are divided to expose the gland.
- During dissection the facial artery and anterior facial vein are ligated and divided. The lingual and hypoglossal nerves are identified and protected. The submandibular duct is identified and divided.

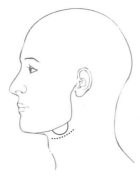

Fig. 8.4   Incision for removal of the submandibular gland.

■ Following removal of the gland the wound is irrigated with saline, haemostasis checked and closure completed after a vacuum drain has been placed.

Post-operative care

■ The drain is maintained until drainage clears (usually 24 to 28 hours)
■ Sutures are removed at between 5 and 7 days

Complications

■ **Facial weakness:** the mandibular branch of the facial nerve is at risk during the procedure. Damage to this branch will result in drooping of the lower lip on the affected side.
■ **Tongue sensation:** damage to the lingual nerve will result in impaired taste and sensation on the affected side.
■ **Tongue movement:** damage to the hypoglossal nerve will result in deviation of the protruded tongue towards the affected side.

Operations on the submandibular duct

Anterior calculi can be removed under local anaesthetic. Traction sutures are used to elevate the duct and stone before cutting down directly onto the stone if this is readily identifiable (Fig. 8.5). When the stone is posteriorly placed the submandibular duct is identified and traced posteriorly to the site of the stone. In operations on the posterior duct it is essential to identify and protect the lingual nerve which crosses the duct in the first molar region

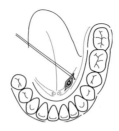

Fig. 8.5   Removal of a submandibular duct stone with stay suture passed under the stone to elevate the tissue and prevent the stone from slipping backwards towards the gland.

Removal of the sublingual gland

Indications

A mucous cyst in the floor of the mouth may arise from the minor salivary glands, but the sublingual gland itself may give rise to a retention cyst (ranula). Superficial cysts are sometimes treated by marsupialisation (i.e. de-roofing), but for a more deeply placed cyst of the gland removal of the whole gland is necessary.

Diagnosis

- Recurrent swelling under the tongue
- Incision or aspiration will confirm the diagnosis and give temporary relief

Aims

Removal of the gland without damage to adjacent structures (the lingual nerve and submandibular duct).

Pre-operative preparation

Patient information and informed consent. Special reference to tongue sensation.

Operating theatre procedure

Instruments required

- Intra-oral soft tissue set (*see* Fig. 4.5)
- Local anaesthetic for infiltration

Anaesthesia

General with naso-tracheal intubation.

Position

Standard for intra-oral procedure.

Preparation of operative site

■ Standard peri-oral preparation
■ Standard head towels

Operative procedure

■ The floor of the mouth may be infiltrated with local anaesthetic and the gland approached via an incision or flap (Fig. 8.6)
■ Stay sutures may be used to improve tongue retraction
■ The sublingual duct and the lingual nerve are identified prior to dissection and delivery of the gland
■ Haemostasis is checked and the wound closed with resorbable sutures

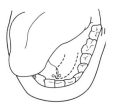

Fig. 8.6   Incision for removal of sublingual gland.

Post-operative care

■ Standard oral hygiene measures
■ Antibiotic cover
■ Analgesia

Complications

■ Damage to the submandibular duct may produce obstruction of the submandibular gland.
■ Damage to the lingual nerve would produce loss of tongue sensation on the affected side.

Minor salivary gland surgery

Mucous retention cyst excision

Indications

The commonest site for a mucocele is the lower lip. Recurrent swelling is typical, sometimes with intermittent discharge of the cyst contents.

Diagnosis

Typically a superficial bluish swelling about 1 cm in diameter.

Aims

Removal of the lesion without damage to adjacent structures.

Pre-operative preparation of the patient

Patient information and informed consent – standard for intra-oral soft tissue procedure. Special reference to lip sensation.

Operating theatre (or clinic) procedure

Instruments required

- Intra-oral soft tissue set (*see* Fig. 4.7)
- Local anaesthetic

Anaesthesia

Usually local anaesthetic.

Position

Standard.

Preparation of operative site

Standard.

Operative procedure

- The lower lip is retracted with some tension and an incision made over the swelling (Fig. 8.7)

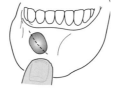

Fig. 8.7 Excision of mucous retention cyst in lower lip.

- Rupture of the cyst often occurs at some stage during the dissection
- The mucous glands at the base of the cyst must be removed to prevent recurrence
- The incision is closed with resorbable sutures

Post-operative care

Standard for intra-oral soft tissue procedure.

Complications

- Recurrence due to incomplete excision of the basal mucous glands
- Sensory deficit on lower lip due to damage to mental nerve fibres which are submucosal in this region

Palatal pleomorphic adenoma excision

Indications

The commonest site for a pleomorphic adenoma of the minor salivary glands is the area of the junction of hard and soft palate. A painless, slow-growing swelling is typical.

Diagnosis

- History and clinical appearance
- Biopsy

Aims

Complete excision of tumour.

Pre-operative preparation

Standard for intra-oral procedure. Informed consent with special reference to palatal dressing or plate, speech and swallowing.

Operating theatre procedure

Instruments

Intra-oral soft tissue set (*see* Fig. 4.5).

Anaesthesia

General, naso-tracheal intubation.

Position

Standard for intra-oral procedure with neck fully extended.

Preparation of operative site

- Standard peri- and intra-oral preparation
- Standard head towels

Operative procedure

- An incision is made around the swelling with a margin of at least 0.5 cm (Fig. 8.8).
- The incision is taken down to bone on the hard palate and the dissection performed subperiostally beneath the tumour. The dissection may need to be extended onto the soft palate.
- The greater palatine artery will usually need to be ligated for a lesion at this site.
- A Whitehead's varnish pack is sewn over the wound, or a dental plate fitted.

Post-operative care

Standard for intra-oral procedure.

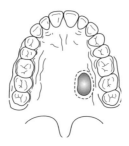

Fig. 8.8   Excision of palatal pleomorphic adenoma.

Complications

- Palatal fistula
- Speech and swallowing difficulties if soft palate involved

Large, long-standing lesions may erode the bone of the hard palate. Excision as described above would produce an oronasal fistula. This may be obturated with a dental plate, or preferably repaired by a palatal rotation flap. Similarly, a large adenoma of the soft palate needing full thickness excision will need suitable repair. Malignant tumours of the minor salivary glands in this area require a partial maxillectomy (*see* Chapter 11, part I).

Summary

The salivary glands may be involved in a wide range of pathological processes, varying from obstruction of a minor salivary gland to a malignant tumour of a major gland. Treatment is mainly surgical and may also range widely between a minor out-patient procedure to a major procedure involving admission, resection and reconstruction.

9

Maxillofacial Trauma

G.D.D. Roberts and C. Roberts

This chapter describes injury to the facial skeleton and soft tissues. Assessment, diagnosis and treatment are covered with emphasis on the details of operative management and after care.

The facial skeleton

The facial skeleton is made up of two parts. The upper portion is fixed immovably to the anterior part of the cranial base. The lower part is the mandible which is freely moveable at the temporomandibular joints. The bony anatomy of the upper facial skeleton is complex and includes the cavities of the mouth (in part), the nose, the sinuses and the orbits. Injury to the facial skeleton and associated soft tissues may therefore involve the organs of sight, respiration and olfaction, mastication and taste. The bones of the facial skeleton are illustrated in Figs A and B in the Introduction.

The soft tissues of the face and mouth are equally complex and injuries to muscles and nerves may occur as well as the more obvious damage to skin and mucosa. The main sensory nerve of the region is the trigeminal (Vth cranial, *see* Introduction, Fig. D). Branches of this nerve in the bony canals in the mandible and malar are especially vulnerable to injury in fractures of these bones. The facial (VIIth cranial) nerve innervates the muscles of facial expression and gives animation to the face (*see* Introduction Fig. E). Its branches are at risk with some facial lacerations and also during surgery for repair of some facial fractures.

Facial injuries are commonplace and may involve the soft tissues, the facial skeleton or both. The commonest causes of facial injury are:

- Assault
- Sporting injury
- Road traffic accident (RTA)

The cause and background of the injury are important as they may influence management. A high velocity RTA implies different forces to those of assault. The wound from a dog bite will usually be contaminated by organisms not normally encountered in human beings. A case of domestic assault may need social worker involvement prior to discharge.

Preliminary assessment

The management of trauma generally is addressed in specific ways according to advanced trauma life support (ATLS) protocols. This is beyond the scope of this book. However, it must be stressed that a thorough general assessment of the injured patient must always take place, if other less obvious serious injuries are not to be overlooked. Specific points should be emphasised in relation to maxillofacial trauma and the well known ABC approach to initial trauma assessment ensures that early priorities are correct.

ABC of trauma

Airway

- Patients with orofacial injuries are at great risk of airway obstruction, especially if not fully conscious, and any problems must be addressed immediately.
- The mouth must be cleared of all blood and debris, identifying broken tooth fragments and dentures.
- Postural aids may be necessary – the recovery position or pulling the jaw forward.
- Mechanical aids may be necessary – artificial airway (e.g. Guedel) or intubation.
- Severe bleeding is unusual in maxillofacial injuries, but nasal packing is occasionally required.
- Tracheostomy is rarely required.

Breathing

After the airway is secured, breathing must be maintained, with ventilation if necessary.

Circulation

The monitoring of vital signs and an estimate of blood loss will allow fluid replacement to be planned.

Head injury

Initially a rapid assessment may be made and patients classified as:

- Alert
- Verbally responding
- Pain responsive
- Unresponsive

Further detail is beyond the scope of this chapter and head injury is best monitored using an agreed points protocol such as the Glasgow coma scale (GCS).

Cerebrospinal fluid (CSF) leak implies a communication into the cranial cavity through the meninges, allowing the escape of CSF. Equally this allows the potential for infection to cause meningitis or cerebral abscess. It is usual to give prophylactic antibiotic cover specifically for this risk. A CSF leak presents as straw coloured fluid from the nose or ear and the diagnosis can be confirmed biochemically, indicating base of skull fracture. CSF escape from the nose indicates anterior cranial fossa fracture, and from the ear indicates middle cranial fossa fracture. All middle third fractures of the maxilla have the potential for CSF leak.

Cervical spine injury

Exclusion of neck injuries is an essential part of the early assessment. Further damage, for example quadriplegia, can be caused by careless movement of patients with neck injuries. Radiography of the cervical spine should exclude bony injury.

Control of pain

Pain relief is an essential part of patient management. It helps to stabilise the patient and relieve some of the stress of trauma. If the patient is likely to need general anaesthesia, discussion with the anaesthetist regarding pain relief is advisable as some drugs may mask observations. In fracture cases immobilisation and fixation will help ease pain.

Protocols for pain relief may be helpful. The use of a patient controlled analgesia (PCA) administration system is helpful in major cases. Pain control drugs may be administered:

- Orally
- Rectally
- Intramuscularly
- Intravenously

A wide range of drugs is available:

- Minor, e.g. paracetamol
- Intermediate, e.g. diclofenac
- Major, e.g. morphine

Control of infection

Infection in relation to maxillofacial injury is not common and this is partly related to the excellent blood supply of the region. Measures to reduce the incidence of infection may be local or general:

- **Local:** wound debridement involves removal of foreign bodies and dead tissue. Because of the good blood supply it is not usually necessary to excise tissue when repairing lacerations unless severely damaged.

- **General:** tetanus protection should be checked; prophylactic antibiotics are often administered for bony injury.

If present, infection should be treated according to established principles:

- Drainage
- Antibiotic therapy following swabs for culture and sensitivity of organisms

Head and neck infections usually respond to:

- Penicillin in various forms
- Cephalosporins
- Metronidazole

Intravenous antibiotics give high blood levels quickly and can later be changed to easier and cheaper oral preparations. Intramuscular drugs are best avoided, if possible, as they are painful to receive and relatively time consuming to give. Normally antibiotics are given for about 5 days, but may be extended to longer periods in special circumstances such as prolonged infection and resistant strains of organisms.

It is important to ascertain if the patient is allergic to any antibiotics or other drugs before initiating therapy. An allergic reaction to any drug, especially penicillin, may develop into life threatening anaphylaxis

History taking

Obtaining the history may be difficult, but is an essential part of the process. Accompanying persons will often be able to provide details, especially if the patient is unable to communicate effectively. It may be appropriate to take the history after a brief preliminary assessment or it may be necessary to wait until after resuscitation.

General physical examination

This examination will be carried out by the receiving casualty officer. Nevertheless, the maxillofacial team must be aware of the potential complications, especially in RTA. All examinations must be confirmed by the team accepting a patient.

Specific examination for maxillofacial trauma

For the purposes of examination and description, the face is divided into three parts:

- **The upper third** consists of the frontal and temporal bones continuous with the cranium.
- **The middle third:**
  - □ Two maxillae – the main bones of the central portion of the midface
  - □ Two zygomas – the main bones of the lateral midface
  - □ Other bones are the nasal and lachrymal, the ethmoids and parts of the sphenoid
- **The lower third** is made up of the mandible which articulates with the base of the skull at the temporomandibular joints.

Examination of the head and neck region should proceed in an organised manner normally starting with the cranium then down the face towards the neck:

- Orbits
- Nasal bones
- Maxilla and mandible, including range of movement, dental occlusion and teeth
- Soft tissues
- Neurological, especially the function of the trigeminal (sensory) and facial (motor) nerves

The signs of fracture are swelling, bruising, pain and deformity.

Special priority must be given to the eyes, which might be difficult to examine because of swelling. Ophthalmic opinion should be sought urgently if there is any suspicion of globe injury.

Radiology

Appropriate and good quality X-rays are essential in the diagnosis and management of maxillofacial injuries and should be carried out as soon as possible, although the patient's condition may prevent this immediately after the examination. The most commonly requested films for facial fractures are:

- **Fractured mandible**
  - □ OPT (orthopantomogram – a rotational tomogram of the jaws)
  - □ PA mandible (posteroanterior view of the mandible)
- **Fractured maxilla or zygoma**
  - □ OM 10° and 30° (occipito-mental views)
  - □ Lateral facial bones

Further special techniques, such as computerised axial tomography (CT scan) and magnetic resonance imaging (MRI), may also be necessary.

Soft tissue injuries

Soft tissue injuries of the face are very common. Prompt and correct management of these injuries is important as delay or poor surgery may adversely affect the outcome, leading to unnecessary disfigurement and dissatisfaction, and possibly to formal complaint or litigation.

Wound healing

Soft tissue injuries cannot be properly managed without an understanding of wound healing. Wound healing occurs by:

- Primary intention
- Secondary intention
- Tertiary or delayed intention – rare due to the excellent blood supply in the head and neck

Primary healing is the best outcome where the wound edges are approximated and the layers heal quickly with minimal scarring. Secondary intention is where there is either skin loss or other separation of wound edges. The healing takes place from the base of the wound, gradually filling the defect but leaving gross scarring. Tertiary or delayed intention implies wound breakdown due to infection or systemic causes with poor healing, leading again to gross scarring. There may be a need in these cases for surgical revision of scars.

Phases of wound healing

Inflammatory phase
Over the first 2 to 3 days, the wound is red and inflamed, with swelling, pain, raised temperature and impaired function. This period is increased with large wounds, infection and the presence of foreign bodies. It is also adversely affected by drugs, e.g. cortisone, by disease, e.g. diabetes and leukaemia, and by the presence of necrotic tissue.

Proliferative phase
This is the growth period for capillaries and fibroblasts creating granulation tissue which eventually becomes new normal tissue. This process is delayed by low oxygen tension due to poor blood supply or anaemia, and also by previous irradiation, malnutritional states and increasing age. This phase takes about 14 days.

Maturation phase
This is a consolidation phase whereby the scar shrinks, becoming white, and the granulations are replaced by normal tissue. This phase is long and

may take up to a year, after which it is fairly safe to assume that this is the final result.

Management

The general principles of trauma management apply. The aetiology and medical history are of importance. A dog bite may be managed differently from an RTA. Physical examination must exclude or diagnose associated injuries.

Examination should include careful charting of facial wounds, including diagrams, which can be important in describing the injuries later, for example in connection with medical reports and litigation. Facial soft tissue injury may present as:

- Lacerations
- Abrasions
- Tissue loss

The aim is to restore function and appearance.

Surgical treatment includes wound toilet or lavage to remove all debris and foreign bodies. Failure to do this prior to formal closure of wounds may cause tattooing, which can cause major facial disfigurement. Primary closure in layers is the treatment of choice, but if there is tissue loss it may be necessary to use a flap or skin graft for repair. These techniques are discussed in the chapter on malignancy. Placing the scar along lines of election will also be discussed in that chapter.

Suturing

- Primary: the first person to suture the patient's wound has the best chance of getting a good result.
- Secondary revision surgery will always be second best to primary surgery. If primary suturing has been inadequate revision will be required.
- The purpose of suturing is to approximate the wound edges and hold them in place until the repair is strong enough to hold the position without them. This period varies in different anatomical sites. If the sutures are too tight, the blood supply may be impaired leading to poor healing. Sutures may cause inflammation and become infected. Sutures may fail from incorrect technique or poor choice of material.
- Wounds are always closed in layers (e.g. muscle, subcutaneous fat and skin). Superficial closure alone will leave dead space beneath the surface which will predispose to wound infection and cause spreading of the scar.

- Initially anatomical landmarks should be sought, especially in irregular and extensive wounds. An example of this is a laceration through the vermilion border of the lip. The first stitch should bring together the vermilion margin on each side of the wound, thus allowing the edges to be matched. If this is not done, the margins may not coincide and a gross disfigurement may be created.

Suture materials for the face

For the skin

- Non-absorbable
  - □ Synthetic – fine monofilament, e.g. polypropylene or polybutester
  - □ Natural – silk has been the natural fibre of choice in the past but nowadays is not popular
- Absorbable – materials such as polydioxanone (PDS) can be used for the face in very young children in an attempt to avoid the need for anaesthesia or sedation for suture removal, but they are slow to resorb.

For deeper tissue (fat, muscle)
Absorbable sutures such as catgut or polyglycolic acid are used.

Intra-oral sutures
These are usually absorbable. The rate of absorption is important.

- Natural – plain catgut lasts 2 to 3 days before losing its inherent strength; chromic catgut lasts approximately 10 days.
- Synthetic sutures e.g. polyglactin, polydioxanone, last longer (1 to 3 months) and usually need to be removed.

Wounds are sometimes held with metal clips instead of sutures. This is only really suitable in areas which are mainly hidden from view and the best example in maxillofacial trauma would be the bicoronal flap mentioned later in this chapter.

The size of the suture is determined by the need to have an acceptable appearance, against the need for strength. The maximum used for facial skin would be 3/0 in areas not seen, such as within the hair line, down to 6/0 for fine suturing in thin tissue around the eyes. Needles are round bodied or cutting, and seamlessly attached to the suture material.

Methods of suturing

Careful tissue handling, elimination of dead space and avoidance of a large mass of suture material are essential requirements. The choices of suture method are:

- Interrupted – individual sutures are equally interspersed along the wound.
- Continuous – the suture is continuous along the wound.
- Subcutaneous or subcuticular – these are buried sutures which may be of both absorbable and non-absorbable material. They may produce less scarring and may be easier to remove.
- Mattress – either horizontal or vertical in four point contact giving more substance to the skin edge contact.

Suture removal is carried out at the chosen time with regard to the factors mentioned above:

- Usually about 3 to 5 days for the face
- 5 to 7 days for the neck
- 7 to 10 days intra-orally

A dedicated post-operative dressing clinic is very useful. Removal of sutures for children is usually best carried out by trained children's nurses. The use of adhesive strips after suture removal may help to support the wound edges for a few days longer.

Patients should be instructed how to look after facial wounds after treatment. Usually they will be asked to wash wounds lightly, but not to bathe or soak for about 10 days. The use of chloromycetin ointment on the wound suture line will help to keep it soft and avoid hard scab formation which is difficult to remove and may delay healing and promote infection. Later use of emollient creams may promote healing and speed up scar resolution slightly.

Follow-up of patients with soft tissue injuries is usual for a year, by which time the scar will have healed and will be permanent, with little further change expected. At this time the decision regarding the need for revision of the scar should be taken. Careful attention to the psychological aspects of care will help the patient to come to terms with any disfigurement. Disfigurement may also be helped by camouflage advice.

Fractures of the facial skeleton

All fractures are classified as simple or compound. Simple fractures are uncomplicated and do not connect with the body surfaces. Compound fractures connect with the surface, that is with skin or mucosa, and are therefore prone to contamination and infection. Other descriptions include comminuted, meaning fragmentation due to extreme violence, and pathological, which indicates the presence of a pathological process, such as a cyst, malignant change or osteoporosis, which has been responsible (at least in part) for the fracture.

Aetiology

The causes fall into four main categories which apply to all facial fractures:

- Accidental
- Assault
- Sporting injury
- Road traffic accident (RTA)

Principles of treatment

Reduction, fixation and immobilisation are the principles of all fracture management.

- Direct fixation involves exposure of the fracture site (intra- or extra-orally) with reduction and fixation of the fracture by plates, screws, pins or wires.
- Open reduction and internal fixation (ORIF) is most commonly carried out using plates. Many maxillofacial plating systems are available with numerous shapes of plate in different thicknesses to suit every situation. A good drill and irrigation system is essential. Instructional courses for ORIF are run by some companies for both surgeons and nurses.
- Indirect fixation involves reducing and immobilising the fracture using eyelet wires, arch bars or splints attached to the teeth. Upper and lower jaws can then be secured to each other by intermaxillary fixation (IMF) using wires or elastics. If there is no direct fixation of the fracture, IMF will be required for the healing period (3 to 6 weeks).
- Restoration of the correct dental occlusion is vital in jaw fracture surgery.

Children

Children may need specific care. They may exhibit a 'greenstick' fracture which only occurs in young bone. The healing capacity is greater and fractures may not need the same level of intervention. Developing teeth may be damaged by the treatment as well as the injury. Condylar fractures may interfere with mandibular growth and must be monitored.

Fractures of the mandible

Mandibular fractures may be:

- Simple
- Compound (almost all fractures in the tooth bearing parts of the mandible are compound into the mouth)
- Comminuted
- Pathological

Fractures may be:

- Unilateral
- Bilateral
- Multiple

According to site, fractures are described as:

- Condylar
- Coronoid
- Angle
- Body
- Symphyseal (midline)
- Parasymphyseal (lateral to the midline)
- Dentoalveolar

(*see* Fig. 9.1).

Diagnosis

- Pain
- Swelling and bruising

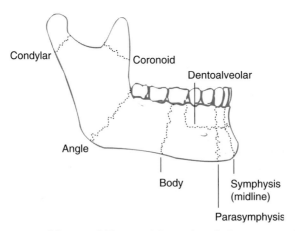

Fig. 9.1 Fractures of the mandible. Condylar and angle fractures are the most common sites.

- Bleeding
- Crepitus caused by movement at the fracture site
- Trismus – limitation of mandibular movement
- Malocclusion – incorrect bite
- Neurodeficit – paraesthesia of the lower lip

During clinical examination, using a good light source, debris is cleared away. Associated soft tissue injury, intra-oral bruising and dental damage may indicate underlying bony injury. Missing teeth should be accounted for as they may have been inhaled.

Investigations

Radiographs:

- Orthopantomogram (OPT)
- Posteroanterior (PA) view of the mandible

Aims

Primary bone healing with full restoration of function and appearance.

Pre-operative preparation of the patient

- Patient information – warnings regarding possibility of IMF, loss of teeth and neurodeficit
- Consent
- Pre-operative anaesthetic assessment
- Standard check list for general anaesthetic
- Ensure X-rays are available

Operating theatre procedure

Instruments required

- Intra-oral set (*see* Fig. 4.5)
- Plating set (*see* Fig. 4. 12)
- Fracture/wiring set (*see* Figs 4.10 and 4.11)
- Drill with irrigation (*see* Fig. 4.14)

Anaesthesia

Usually general anaesthetic with naso-tracheal intubation and throat pack.

Position

Standard for intra-oral procedure.

Preparation of operative site

■ Standard peri-oral
■ Standard head towels and drapes for oral procedure

Operative procedure

The example given is for a fracture of the body of the mandible treated by open reduction and internal fixation (ORIF) using plates and temporary IMF (Fig. 9.2).

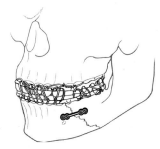

Fig. 9.2   Fracture of the body of the mandible fixed with a miniplate after the application of temporary IMF using arch bars. The IMF is removed at the end of the procedure.

■ Eyelet wires or arch bars are applied to the teeth
■ An intra-oral incision is made and a muco-periosteal flap reflected to fully expose the fracture site
■ The fracture site is thoroughly debrided and irrigated
■ IMF is established and the reduction of the fracture checked and adjusted if necessary
■ A suitable plate is contoured and fixed across the fracture site. The dental occlusion is checked throughout the plating procedure
■ The wound is again thoroughly irrigated and closed with resorbable sutures
■ The IMF is released and the dental occlusion checked again
■ The throat pack is removed and the pharynx cleared by suction
■ Petroleum jelly is applied to the lips

Not all fractures of the mandible need operative treatment. Undisplaced fractures and most unilateral condylar fractures may be managed conservatively. Simple fractures may be managed by IMF without open reduction and direct fixation, and with a suitable patient may be carried out under local anaesthetic. With this method however, the jaws will need to remain immobilised and fixed together for up to 6 weeks to allow fracture healing.

Temporary IMF does not always need to be applied prior to open reduction of a fracture as it is sometimes possible to manually reduce the fracture while plating takes place. Where intra-oral access to the fracture is difficult, plating may be carried out through an extra-oral or percutaneous approach.

Post-operative care

Immediate

If IMF in wire form is used, there is a specific need for special care of the patient with respect to the airway. This is usually managed in high dependency or intensive care units. A special wire cutting kit is needed, with attention given to suction and patient positioning. Prevention and management of vomiting may be required.

Intermediate

General care of the post-operative patient is not within the scope of this chapter. Specific points with maxillofacial injuries are:

- Posture
- Prevention of infection (prophylactic antibiotics)
- Analgesia and sedation
- Oral hygiene instruction
- Feeding and nutrition especially if IMF is used
- Post-operative radiographs

Late

Later management includes determining the period of immobilisation, removal of fixation and testing repair strength, adjustment of dental occlusion, mobilisation of mandible, checking damaged teeth and gums, and checking the progress of any neurodeficit.

Out-patient follow-up and written communications and instructions are essential.

Complications

- Wound infection
- Bony malunion and non-union of the fracture

■ Neurodeficit of the facial and trigeminal nerves may occur and must be monitored, e.g. numbness of lip or tongue. (Primary or secondary repair of damaged nerves may be possible).

Dislocation of the jaw (*see also* Chapter 10)

Injury to the jaw may occur without fracture. Dislocation of the jaw is a relatively common complaint, and may occur as a result of injury or spontaneously. The mandibular condyle is displaced from the glenoid fossa in the base of the skull, rupturing the capsule of the joint. The displacement can be confirmed radiologically.

Unilateral dislocation will make it impossible for the patient to bring the teeth together in the correct dental occlusion, with the jaw deviated markedly away from the affected side. Bilateral dislocation prevents the patient from closing the mouth fully, due to premature contact of the posterior teeth.

Immediate reduction is required to avoid further damage and discomfort. This involves downwards and backwards manual pressure on the posterior teeth and jaw, guiding the condyle(s) over the articular eminence, back into the glenoid fossa (Fig. 9.3). The use of local or general anaesthesia may be required, but reduction can usually be achieved with gentle but firm pressure without anaesthesia.

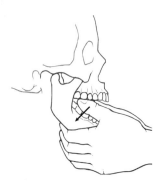

Fig. 9.3 Reduction of dislocated mandible. The force applied is predominantly downwards and backwards.

Fractures of the maxilla

Classification (Fig. 9.4)

■ Le Fort I: fracture line above maxillary teeth, horizontally separating the teeth and palate from the rest of the midface.

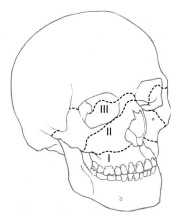

Fig. 9.4   The Le Fort fracture lines in the upper facial skeleton.

■ Le Fort II: pyramidal fracture through orbital rim to base of nose, separating nose, palate and teeth from the rest of the midface.
■ Le Fort III: high level horizontal fracture through lateral orbital margins, separating the whole midface from the cranium.

Rene Le Fort, a Frenchman, devised the classification following his research in the post-mortem room during the nineteenth century. He dropped heavy weights onto the faces of the cadavers and noticed how the resultant fractures fell into the three categories. In practice, severe injuries are frequently a combination of fracture at different levels (Fig. 9.5).

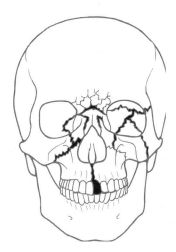

Fig. 9.5   Severe, comminuted fracture of the upper facial skeleton with fractures at all Le Fort levels.

Clinical examination

The examination includes the general and specific principles already discussed. Particular points for the maxilla are as follows:

■ Mobility of maxilla
■ Occlusal derangement – often gagging on posterior teeth
■ Periorbital swelling and bruising
■ Intra-oral bruising in the upper buccal sulci and soft palate
■ 'Cracked cup' sound when teeth are percussed
■ Split palate in the midline
■ Subconjunctival haemorrhage
■ CSF leak from nose
■ Neurodeficit – paraesthesia of the upper lip and cheeks
■ Diplopia
■ Deformity – general 'dish face' appearance and orbital rim step deformity

Tell-tale signs: **swelling, bruising, tenderness, deformity** and **mobility**.

Treatment

Principles of treatment are as for any fracture as described before.

■ Treatment is usually by ORIF. Access may be intra-oral for low level fractures. Higher level Le Fort II and III fractures may require an infra-orbital or lateral orbital approach.
■ Complicated cases may require a bicoronal flap whereby the scalp is brought forward over the face to provide the access needed.
■ In comminuted cases, indirect fixation using halo or box frame methods may rarely be employed.
■ IMF may also be used in some circumstances.

Post-operative care and complications

The same principles apply as described for the fractured mandible.

Fractures of the zygomatic complex

Fracture of the zygoma (malar or cheek bone) is one of the commonest of all facial fractures. It can be difficult to recognise and may be missed initially, especially when there is facial swelling and minimal displacement. The bone structure is complex.

The zygoma is attached to the other midface bones in four places as follows:

- Frontal bone at the fronto-zygomatic suture (F-Z suture)
- The temporal bone at the zygomatic arch
- The maxilla at the orbital margin
- The maxilla again at the lateral wall of the maxillary antrum

These four sutures or joining points are often the sites of fracture of the zygomatic complex and are best confirmed by 10° and 30° occipitomental (OM) X-ray views. Detailed classification of the bony displacement exists, but the fractured zygoma is usually driven inwards and downwards (Fig. 9.6).

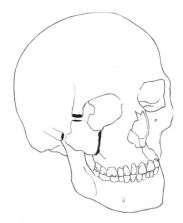

Fig. 9.6 Fracture of the zygoma. The displacement is mainly downwards and inwards.

Diagnosis and clinical examination

History and examination follow the described general form for maxillo-facial injuries. Particular points for the zygoma are:

- Subconjunctival haemorrhage – also seen in maxillary fractures
- Deformity
  - Orbital – step palpable on orbital rim
  - Arch – may present as dimple in cheek
  - Flattening of cheek – may be initially masked by swelling
- Infra-orbital paraesthesia/anaesthesia
- Diplopia
- Trismus – impaction of fracture on coronoid process of mandible may inhibit mobility of the mandible

Ophthalmological opinion is sought as an emergency for patients with signs of damage to the eye, and later for those with diplopia. There may be early or late bleeding from the nostril due to bleeding into the maxillary antrum. Patients should be warned not to blow the nose as the increase in pressure can force air into the tissues causing surgical emphysema. This can be recognised by palpation of crepitus or 'crackling' of the soft tissues around the orbit.

Treatment

Management of the zygomatic complex injury may involve surgery. However surgery may not be necessary for minimally displaced fractures, and may even be contra-indicated in some situations. If the other eye is blind it may be better to leave the fracture untreated. Medically compromised patients may be better left if the surgery is only to improve appearance. It is a matter of weighing advantage against possible complications such as blindness. A few days' delay may help the decision.

Surgery

■ Closed reduction: the Gillies closed elevation is a very effective way of reducing many zygomatic fractures. There are other methods of closed reduction including the Poswillo hook. The success of closed reduction depends on the inherent stability of the fracture, as there is no specific fixation.
■ ORIF is necessary for unstable fractures. Microplates are usually employed around the orbital margins, mainly at the infra-orbital margin or F-Z suture.
■ Orbital floor injuries are repaired by repositioning the orbital contents from an infra-orbital approach and covering the floor defect with a graft. The graft may be autologous from the patient in the form of bone or cartilage from the skull and ear respectively, or synthetic material such as silicone (Silastic) or polydioxanone (PDS) which is resorbable.

An example is given for a zygomatic fracture treated by elevation and ORIF.

Pre-operative preparation of the patient

■ Patient information – warning regarding skin incision, hair shaving and neurodeficit
■ Consent
■ Pre-operative anaesthetic assessment
■ Standard check list for general anaesthetic
■ Ensure X-rays are available

Operating theatre procedure

Instruments required

- Intra-oral set (*see* Fig. 4.5)
- Extra-oral soft tissue set
- Fracture set (*see* Fig. 4.10)
- Plating set (*see* Fig. 4.12)
- Drill with irrigation (*see* Fig. 4.14)

Anaesthesia

General with orotracheal intubation and throat pack.

Position

Standard with moderate head up tilt with the head turned to the opposite side.

Preparation of operative site

- Hair may be shaved or parted in the temporal area
- Chloramphenicol ointment to the eye
- Standard head towels leaving the upper face exposed on the operative side

Operative procedure

- An incision is made above the hairline in the temporal area and deepened to the level of the deep temporal fascia.
- The fascia is incised, a zygomatic elevator is inserted beneath the fascia, passed down under the zygoma, and the bone elevated into the correct position while the assistant steadies the patient's head (Fig. 9.7).
- If the fracture is adequately reduced and stable, further treatment is not required and the temporal incision is closed.
- If not stable, ORIF is necessary. There are three sites for this:
  - □ The fronto-zygomatic region
  - □ The infra-orbital rim
  - □ The malar buttress (intra-oral)
- An incision is made in the appropriate area and the fracture site exposed by subperiosteal dissection.
- Fixation is by plates (usually) or wires and the fracture must be properly reduced and supported using the zygomatic elevator while the plate is contoured and fixed.

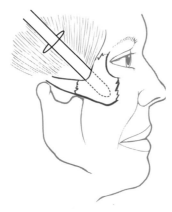

Fig. 9.7   Elevation of fracture of zygoma. Elevator passes down beneath the fracture, through skin and fascial incisions.

- Wounds are irrigated, checked for haemostasis and closed in layers.
- The throat pack is removed and the pharynx cleared by suction.

Post-operative care and complications

The same principles apply as described for the fractured mandible. Care of the eyes is paramount and should be checked regularly after injuries to the midface. An eye observation chart is shown in Fig. 9.8.

Orbital floor injury

Orbital floor injury is a component of all zygomatic fractures, but may occur in isolation without zygomatic fracture – the 'blow-out' fracture (Fig. 9.9).

Significant disruption of the orbital floor will allow orbital soft tissue to herniate into the maxillary antrum, producing the following signs and symptoms:

- Enophthalmos – sunken eye, due to loss of orbital contents
- Diplopia – due to entrapment of the inferior rectus and inferior oblique muscles
- Paraesthesia of the cheek and upper lip caused by injury to the infra-orbital nerve in the orbital floor

Investigations

- Orthoptic assessment of eye movement
- Radiographic – occipito-mental view may show classical 'tear drop' appearance of orbital soft tissue herniating into the maxillary antrum

NURSING EYE OBSERVATION CHART

Name of Patient . . . . Hospital Number . . . .

Consultant . . . .

The signs and symptoms of a retrobulbar haemorrhage are one or more of the following:

1. Orbital pain
2. Decreasing vision
3. Increasing proptosis
4. Decreasing pupil response
5. Dilated pupil

This condition can lead to irreversible blindness. If suspected the duty maxillofacial surgeon should be informed *immediately* as prompt action may be required.

Please assess:
1. Orbital pain as present (✔) or not (✗)
2. Visual acuity as normal (✔)
   reduced (R)
   absent (✗)
3. Proptosis as present (✔) or not (✗)
4. Pupil response to light   Equality   e = equal
   (1) = reacts   u = unequal
   (2) = sluggish
   (3) = no reaction
5. Pupil size

1 mm	·
2 mm	•
3 mm	•
4 mm	●
5 mm	●
6 mm	●
7 mm	●

¼ hourly for first 2 hours		Orbital pain (✔ ✗)		Visual acuity (✔ R ✗)		Proptosis (✔ ✗)		Pupil response (1–3)		(e u)	Pupil size (1–7)	
Date	Time	R	L	R	L	R	L	R	L	equal	R	L

½ hourly for first 2 hours		Orbital pain (✔ ✗)		Visual acuity (✔ R ✗)		Proptosis (✔ ✗)		Pupil response (1–3)		(e u)	Pupil size (1–7)	
Date	Time	R	L	R	L	R	L	R	L	equal	R	L

Fig. 9.8 Nursing eye observation chart.

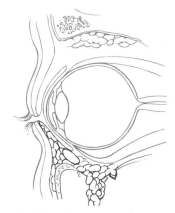

Fig. 9.9   Fracture of the orbital floor showing prolapse of orbital fat into the maxillary antrum.

■ Computerised tomography (CT) is routine for suspected orbital floor injury

Fractures of the nose

History and examination as before. Signs of simple nasal fracture are:

■ Pain, bruising and swelling
■ Deviation of nasal septum
■ Nasal deformity
■ Epistaxis
■ Obstruction of nasal airway

Treatment

Closed manipulation and splintage is usually adequate for most nasal fractures. Submucous resection of the nasal septum (SMR) may be required.

Fractures of the naso-ethmoidal complex (Fig. 9.10)

This is a severe and complicated injury and may be part of a Le Fort II or III fracture. The bones involved are:

■ Nasal
■ Frontal
■ Lacrimal
■ Ethmoid

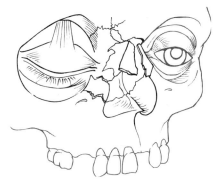

Fig. 9.10   Nasoethmoidal fracture with bony comminution and disruption of the insertion of medial canthal ligaments.

Displacement of the medial canthal ligaments which are attached to the lacrimal bones causes telecanthus (increased width between the eyes). The signs are those of the midface injury with, in addition, nasal deformity and depression of the nasal bridge together with increased intercanthal distance. The diagnosis should be confirmed with appropriate X-rays which will include CT scan.

Treatment

Treatment will include any head injury management and infection prophylaxis. The aim is to accurately reduce, stabilise and fix the bony fragments and the canthal ligaments by ORIF using a bicoronal flap approach or by local flaps. Wires or microplates are used to restore the anatomy.

Craniofacial fractures

These injuries are combined fractures of the midface and cranium. They are complex and may require referral to the craniofacial team and involve neurosurgery. Careful assessment is necessary. If the patient is to be transferred, this can only be done if initial assessment and resuscitation allows for safe transfer. A nurse or doctor may have to accompany the patient during transfer to another unit.

Treatment

Management of this complex injury requires wide access with a bicoronal flap and ORIF to reconstruct the craniofacial anatomy.

Dentoalveolar trauma

Trauma to the teeth and surrounding alveolar bone is usually caused by falls, assaults, RTAs and sporting accidents. As with other facial injuries it is important to know the full background to the incident. The majority of dental injuries occur during early childhood, coinciding with learning to walk and increased independent mobility. These injuries may be relatively minor or associated with other more serious injuries.

If the patient is seen in hospital, initial treatment must be followed through by the general dental practitioner who must be made aware of the situation as soon as possible.

History

- The location of the incident is important – a clean environment such as a swimming pool is less likely to have caused contamination than a football pitch.
- The timing of the incident is important – the earlier the treatment the better the prognosis, especially for an avulsed tooth.
- Any loss of consciousness indicating a head injury must be noted.
- A thorough medical history is necessary including the tetanus status of the patient.

Examination

Particular points in relation to dentoalveolar trauma are:

- Tooth mobility and displacement
- Missing teeth or tooth fragments which could have been inhaled or embedded in soft tissue
- Alveolar fracture
- Malocclusion
- Soft tissue injury

Investigations

X-rays for root fracture, alveolar fracture and embedded tooth fragments.

Aims of early management

- Control pain
- Protect tooth pulp
- Suture lacerations
- Splint teeth

Antibiotics, tetanus prophylaxis and antibacterial mouthwash may also be required.

Non-accidental injury (NAI)

When young children are involved, the possibility of an NAI should always be considered. In these cases the injury may not correlate with the parent's account of the incident. There may be a delay between the time the incident happened and the presentation for treatment. Bruising of differing ages, and tears of the labial fraenum are other clues. If NAI is suspected social services must be contacted.

Injuries to primary teeth

Management is planned with the health of the permanent successor in mind. Crown and root fractures are rare because of the elasticity of the alveolar bone, therefore the most common injuries are loosening or displacement of the teeth. The management of each injury type is as follows:

- **Subluxation** (loosening) – reassurance, soft diet and analgesia.
- **Luxation** (displacement) – extraction or no treatment depending on displacement. The tooth may be manually repositioned if it interferes with the occlusion.
- **Intrusion** (displacement further into the socket) – this injury requires no treatment and the tooth may re-erupt.
- **Extrusion** (displacement further out of the socket) – these teeth are usually extracted.
- **Avulsion** (displacement completely out of the socket) – primary teeth are not replanted.
- **Crown fracture** – treatment depends on co-operation of the child (see permanent teeth).
- **Root fracture** – if there is little mobility and no displacement, no treatment is necessary; if the coronal portion of the fractured tooth is mobile or displaced, it is extracted leaving the apical root fragment in situ.

Injuries to permanent teeth

Trauma to permanent teeth most commonly results in crown fractures. Root fractures and avulsion are less common.

The site of the fracture is important in determining what treatment is necessary.

Crown fractures

- Enamel only – any sharp edges are smoothed
- Enamel and dentine – the dentine is protected with a dressing
- Enamel and dentine and pulp – the pulp is protected with a dressing

Root fractures

- Apical third – no treatment is required
- Middle third – the tooth is splinted for 8 to 12 weeks
- Coronal third – both portions of the fractured tooth are extracted
- Vertical (longitudinal) – the fragments are extracted

Tooth displacement

- **Subluxation** – no treatment may be necessary if mobility is minimal, but the tooth is splinted for 1 to 2 weeks if mobile.
- **Luxation** – the tooth is manually repositioned and splinted for 2 to 3 weeks.
- **Intrusion** – no immediate treatment is necessary. Teeth with immature roots may re-erupt, but teeth with fully formed roots will require orthodontic extrusion.
- **Extrusion** – the tooth is repositioned manually and splinted for 1 to 2 weeks.

Avulsion

A tooth that has been knocked completely out of its socket requires immediate attention. The treatment of choice is immediate re-implantation by whoever is available at the scene. The prognosis is good if this is done within the hour. An avulsed tooth is best stored in saliva, normal saline or milk and handled minimally. If it is contaminated, the tooth is gently washed in saline and then replaced into the socket. The tooth should be splinted in position for one week and further management is usually undertaken by the general dental practitioner.

Methods of splinting teeth

- **Direct splints:**
  - Acid etch composite with or without orthodontic wire
  - Metal foil temporarily cemented to the teeth
- **Indirect splints:** removable plastic splints temporarily cemented to the teeth. Indirect splints are laboratory made, and dental impressions are needed for their construction

The above account details the immediate and early treatment of traumatised teeth, but long term follow-up is important and normally undertaken by the patient's general dental practitioner. Late complications of trauma to teeth are:

- Pulp necrosis leading to abscess formation and in immature teeth, cessation of root development
- Root resorption

Alveolar fracture

The alveolus is the part of the jaw which contains and supports the teeth. Fractures of the alveolus may be associated with dental trauma as described earlier, as well as with more severe bony fractures of the facial skeleton. Management involves splinting, using the teeth adjacent to the fracture site for 3 to 4 weeks, but if the tooth socket is comminuted, this is increased to 6 to 8 weeks. In addition, larger fragments may need fixation with direct plating.

Summary

Accurate diagnosis and early treatment are essential for rapid return of normal function. Modern techniques of internal fixation will often shorten the patient's stay in hospital and lead to a speedier rehabilitation. The nurses' role especially in relation to operative treatment and after care is paramount.

10

The Temporomandibular Joint

R.P. Juniper

This chapter describes the normal anatomy and function of the temporomandibular joint (TMJ) followed by an account of its disorders. A detailed description is given of the diagnosis and treatment of the commonest TMJ disorder (facial arthromyalgia). This condition is treated conservatively in virtually all cases and patient communication is of the utmost importance. Conditions requiring surgery are relatively uncommon, but are covered individually in terms of the pre-operative preparation of the patient, the operating theatre procedure and aftercare.

Anatomy and physiology

The mandible articulates with the base of the skull through two temporomandibular joints (TMJs). For the mouth to open symmetrically and normally, both joints have to be able to move equally and without pain or impediment. The normal TMJ allows the mouth to open between 45 and 55 mm as measured at the incisor teeth, and allows for about 10 mm movement of the chin each side of the midline (lateral excursion). The TMJ is unique amongst the joints of the body and behaves quite differently from any other, as it has to be lax enough to allow the complex free movements during speech, yet rigid enough to allow powerful incising, tearing and crushing of food. The various functions are achieved through a combination of an intricate organisation of ligaments, a meniscus which moves in a very specific way, and complex neuromuscular control.

The TMJ is made up of a condyle, the most proximal part of the mandible, which articulates with the glenoid fossa and articular eminence, a part of the base of the skull (Fig. 10.1). To facilitate the mixture of rotation and sliding of the condyle against the bones of the base of the skull, the TMJ is divided into two separate joint spaces by a fibrous meniscus. The upper joint space allows for sliding movements, while the lower allows for rotation. (Fig. 10.2). Maximum forward movement of the condyle on opening the mouth or moving the chin to one side is about 15 mm. As this happens, the meniscus moves forwards only 8 mm. It functions rather like the slide on a filing cabinet drawer, allowing supported movement beyond the confines of the true joint itself.

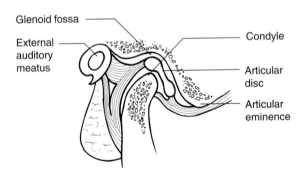

Fig. 10.1   Temporomandibular joint (closed).

The TMJ is supported and moved by the muscles of mastication. The main closing muscles are the temporal, masseter and medial pterygoid, and the opening muscles are the lateral pterygoid attached to the condylar neck, and a series of muscles attached behind the point of the chin, the predominant one of which is the digastric. Each joint is stabilised during

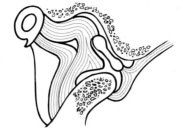

Fig. 10.2   Temporomandibular joint (open).

chewing by the upper part of the lateral pterygoid. As the mandible is one bone with a joint at each end, the muscles of both sides are active in all chewing movements, sometimes to produce power, at other times to produce stability.

It is not surprising that the complex control mechanisms sometimes go wrong.

Disorders of the TMJ

There are various disorders of the TMJ which require treatment, but few require surgery. Growth disorders, either too much growth (hyperplasia) or too little (hypoplasia), which lead to jaw deformity do require surgery without preliminary conservative measures. The same applies to ankylosis, where the mandible becomes fused to the base of the skull, or to tumours which involve the various parts of the joint.

Osteoarthritis and rheumatoid arthritis affect the TMJs less commonly than other joints and are usually managed conservatively. The most common condition, facial arthromyalgia (TMJ dysfunction), seldom requires surgery and should be treated conservatively for months or years before surgery should be considered. When all other treatments have failed and there is a definite indication from existing evidence that the patient is likely to be improved by surgery, then, and then only should surgery be offered.

Facial arthromyalgia (TMJ dysfunction)

A syndrome of clicking, pain and limitation of opening has been known by various names – TMJ dysfunction, myofascial pain dysfunction. A more descriptive term is now favoured – facial arthromyalgia. The symptoms can range from a minor click to a debilitating pain. In its varying forms it is a very common condition affecting up to 25% of the population, with a female/male predominance of up to 5:1. Most patients present at the age of 15 to 25 years, although a few will complain of trouble up to the age of about 45. Beyond this age the condition is uncommon.

History

No specific cause is generally identifiable for this condition, but there may be a history of trauma, such as a blow to the jaw or a wide yawn. This may lead to an acute pain with limitation of jaw movement. A painless click or joint noise may follow and some months or years later, a further episode may occur. The pain may become severe at the limit of opening and the click may cease. Further exacerbations may follow after an inadvertent wide yawn, or a prolonged visit to a dental practitioner.

However, the condition often arises without a history of trauma, frequently at times of stress: there is often some joint pain, but mainly an ache felt in the muscles of mastication. Simple analgesics reduce the pain but do not abolish it and, in a few patients, the discomfort is so severe and prolonged that enjoyment of life is impossible. Many patients will be found to have habits which overload the joints and muscles, such as bruxing (grinding the teeth at night) and clenching the teeth in response to stress. Other significant habits are nail biting and lip biting. One side tends to be affected predominantly. Rarely younger patients may present with very severe acute symptoms which are incapacitating. As stress is an important factor in the condition, consideration must be given to the whole patient, not just to the site of the pain. Causes for stress, such as approaching examinations and social problems, should be sought.

Examination

The condyles can be palpated just in front of the ears and may be tender or a click or grating feeling (crepitus) felt. The muscles of mastication, particularly the masseter, may be tender when the teeth are clenched. Opening of the mouth will be restricted and the chin may deviate to one side.

Treatment

If the pain is severe and persistent analgesics should be taken as required until relief is achieved using methods as described below. Most analgesics help, but the non-steroidal anti-inflammatory analgesics (NSAIDs) such as ibuprofen are the most effective. These are helpful in the short term to reduce the pain, but patients should be warned about the possibility of gastric irritation, particularly in long-term use. It is important to realise that these drugs only cause a suppression of symptoms, perhaps allowing the physical component of the condition to recover.

At least 90% of patients suffering TMJ dysfunction respond to conservative treatment. Explanation as to the cause of the pain helps the patient to identify parafunctional habits, such as teeth clenching or nail biting, and to eradicate them. An explanatory leaflet (Information leaflet No 11) and a simple exercise regimen (Information leaflet No 12) have been found most beneficial. Causes of stress should be identified and eliminated

PATIENT INFORMATION LEAFLET No 11

ORAL and MAXILLOFACIAL SURGERY DEPARTMENT

TEMPOROMANDIBULAR JOINT PROBLEMS

Problems related to the temporomandibular (jaw) joint (TMJ) are common and usually involve one or more of the following symptoms:

1. Pain related to the jaw joint, or in the jaw muscles.
2. Clicking or locking of the jaw.
3. Stiffness.

In addition there may be a sensation of fullness or buzzing in the ears.

The pain which is aching in quality may be stress related and many patients also suffer from other problems such as headache or lower back pain.

There is generally no specific cause for the problem, but symptoms may sometimes follow an event which places some strain on the jaw joint, such as an inadvertent yawn or a visit to the dentist.

Most jaw joint problems improve with treatment and rest and do not indicate a serious underlying problem such as arthritis. Clicking is caused by the cartilage in the joint slipping slightly out of position.

In addition to the treatment which may be prescribed, the following points may prove helpful:

1. Eat soft food and avoid tough meat, French bread, etc.
2. Cut apples and hard fruit or vegetables into small pieces.
3. Stifle yawns and avoid wide mouth opening.
4. Do not bite your nails or lips, or chew pencils.
5. Do not chew gum or chewy sweets.

PATIENT INFORMATION LEAFLET No 12

ORAL and MAXILLOFACIAL SURGERY DEPARTMENT

EXERCISES TO IMPROVE THE FUNCTION OF THE TEMPOROMANDIBULAR (JAW) JOINT AND THE MUSCLES OF MASTICATION

The purpose of the exercise is to prevent clicking of the jaw joint and to strengthen the muscles which pull the jaw backwards. This in turn will relax the muscles which close the mouth, and will prevent those muscles which pull the jaw forward and to one side from functioning. The jaw joint will act more as a hinge and this will take strain off it.

Set aside two five-minute periods each day at a time when you are relaxed and have nothing on your mind. One good time is just before you are going to bed, and another perhaps when you get home from work. Sit upright on a chair and carry out the following manoeuvres.

- Close your mouth on your back teeth, resting the tip of your tongue on your palate just behind the upper front teeth.
- Run the tip of your tongue backwards onto the soft palate as far back as it will go, keeping your teeth together.
- Force the tongue back to maintain contact with the soft palate, and slowly open your mouth until you feel your tongue just being pulled away from it. Do not try to open your mouth further. Keep it in this position for five seconds, and then close your mouth. Relax for five seconds.
- Repeat this manoeuvre slowly over the next five minutes in a firm but relaxed fashion.

As you open your mouth you should feel tension in the muscles at the back of your jaw and beneath your chin. For the first few times you do the exercise you should check in front of a mirror that the lower teeth move vertically downwards and do not deviate even slightly from side to side. If the exercise is being carried out correctly, there will be neither clicks nor noise from the joints – if there is, you must be making some error when carrying out the exercise.

▶

PATIENT INFORMATION LEAFLET No 12 *continued*

Do this exercise no more than the recommended amount for the first week. Initially it may seem to make your pain worse, but this will be as a result of the unaccustomed exercise. Thereafter, do the exercise as often as you can and this will help to strengthen the ligaments around your jaw joints and rest the muscles which close your mouth.

If the exercise is carried out correctly and regularly over a two or three week period, you will retrain your muscles so that your jaw opens and closes smoothly without clicks or jerks, and any pain you have been experiencing will subside.

REMEMBER

- Never bite your fingernails
- Never bite your lower lip
- Avoid biting on your front teeth
- Keep your upper and lower teeth apart when at rest

if possible. If required, further conservative treatment is aimed at reducing muscle hyperactivity. There are two main approaches to this stage:

Appliance therapy
Appliances worn at night, clipped on to the teeth, help many people suffering arthromyalgia. There are many different designs of removable appliance, some clipped to the upper and some to the lower teeth. They are all thought to act by evening out the bite and balancing the tone in the muscles of mastication. They may act too by reducing muscle hyper-activity during sleep. They are used for a few months, mainly at night, and can give considerable relief to a group of patients.

Drug therapy
The tricyclic drugs are of considerable benefit. These drugs, often used for depression, are most successful with many patients, given in small doses, usually at night. They act to reduce anxiety, improve sleep patterns so reducing bruxism, and may function as a centrally acting analgesic.

Where the above regimens fail, or where the patient has had intractable pain over a number of years with failed conservative treatment, then there may be benefit in surgery, after suitable investigation. A preliminary, and sometimes an alternative to surgery, is arthrocentesis, particularly where there is predominant joint pain, as opposed to muscle pain.

Arthrocentesis

(This procedure may also be carried out via the arthroscope – arthroscopy *see below*.)

Aims

To remove inflammatory substances and break down adhesions. The opportunity may be taken to insert anti-inflammatory agents into the joint.

Pre-operative preparation of the patient

- Patient information: this may be in the form of a handout. The essential information for the patient is that the procedure is carried out under local anaesthesia as an out-patient and involves the insertion of two needles into the TMJ through which fluid passes to irrigate the joint. The local anaesthetic might cause temporary facial weakness and an eye patch may need to be worn for a few hours. Some swelling and pain may occur, usually controlled by NSAIDs.
- Consent.

Procedure

Instruments required

- Local anaesthetic
- Instruments for arthrocentesis:
    - ☐ Marking pen and Bonney's blue
    - ☐ Ruler
    - ☐ 2 × 21G needles
    - ☐ 2 × 50 ml Luerlock syringes
    - ☐ Three-way tap
    - ☐ Long extension set
    - ☐ Op-site 18 × 30 (Smith & Nephew) – 2 if bilateral
    - ☐ Discarda pad
    - ☐ 500 ml Hartmann's solution
    - ☐ Ear plug (cut from sponge)
    - ☐ Kidney dish (to collect fluid)
    - ☐ Drugs to insert after arthrocentesis (according to surgeon's wishes)

Position of the patient

The procedure is carried out on a couch or dental chair in the horizontal position. The head is turned away from the operating side.

Preparation of the operative site

- Skin preparation (the hair is not shaved)
- Sterile towels may be used
- A kidney dish to collect irrigation fluid is placed in the nape of the neck with an absorbent pad beneath it

Operative procedure

- Local anaesthetic is given over and into the joint.
- Two 21G needles are inserted into the joint. The irrigation fluid is injected through a cannula into the posterior needle to flow out through the anterior one. A cannula may also be used on the second needle to collect the irrigant.
- At the end of the procedure an anti-inflammatory agent may be washed through the joint.

Post-operative care

- Temporary facial weakness may follow the procedure for the duration of the local anaesthetic and an eye patch may be required
- Analgesia

Surgery

A range of procedures may be carried out. Arthroscopy is primarily diagnostic, but therapeutic procedures can be performed through the arthroscope. Open surgery (arthrotomy) is less commonly indicated, and major procedures, such as condylectomy and joint replacement, are carried out only rarely.

Arthroscopy

Aims

Arthroscopy is primarily diagnostic and allows identification of abnormalities of the joint lining, articular disc and joint surfaces. Treatment can also be given via the arthroscope.

Pre-operative preparation of the patient

- Patient information: this may be in the form of a handout. The operation is carried out via tiny incisions or punctures just in front of the ear through which a miniature telescope is inserted into the joint for inspection and treatment. The patient should be warned of pain and swelling immediately post-operatively, with difficulty in opening the mouth. Very occasionally, haematoma may occur.

■ Consent.
■ Standard check list for general anaesthetic.
■ Hair will need to be shaved in the sideburn area only.

Operating theatre procedure

Instruments required

■ 1:100 000 adrenaline solution in saline for skin and joint infiltration (optional)
■ Instruments for arthroscopy
   □ Marking pen and Bonney's blue
   □ Ruler
   □ 2 × 21G needles
   □ 2 × 50 ml Luerlock syringes
   □ Three-way tap
   □ Long extension set
   □ Op-site 18 × 30 (Smith & Nephew) – 2 if bilateral – with elliptical hole cut in middle to take pinna
   □ TURP drape
   □ Irrigation pouch (1016 3M) – 2 if bilateral
   □ 15 blade
   □ Yankeur sucker end and tubing
   □ Discarda pad
   □ 500 ml Hartmann's solution
   □ 1 ml 1:1000 adrenaline
   □ Jug
   □ Ear plug (cut from sponge)
   □ Camera
   □ Camera lead cover

Autoclaved
   □ Blunt probe (straight)
   □ Blunt probe (curved)
   □ 3 × shaped knives
   □ Mason's gag (covered jaws to protect teeth)

Cidexed
   □ Arthroscope
   □ Light lead
   □ 2 × trocar (1 × blunt, 1 × sharp)
   □ 2 × cannulae
   □ 2 × switching sticks

□ Touhey needle
□ Bipolar probe
□ 0 Prolene (8434 without needle)

Anaesthesia

Naso-tracheal intubation with the tube running over the forehead and fixed with adhesive tape.

Position

Standard, with the head supported and turned away from the operating side.

Preparation of the operative site

- Skin preparation
- Standard head towels prepared to expose the side of the face and ear
- Adhesive drape with an oval hole 6 × 4 cm for the pinna
- Plug of plastic foam is inserted in the ear

Operative procedure

- The skin is marked by a line joining the outer canthus of the eye with the midpoint of the tragus. A second mark is made 10 mm in front of the midpoint of the tragus, 2 mm below the line (Fig. 10.3).
- Normal saline is injected into the upper joint space at the mark using a 21G needle on a 2 ml syringe and movement of the mandible noted (to ensure that the saline is in the correct position).
- A second needle is inserted into the joint space approximately 10 mm anterior to the first to allow saline to run through and out of the joint.
- The first needle is removed and a stab incision made at its entry point.
- 1 ml of saline is injected through the second needle to expand the joint and a trocar and cannula inserted into the joint along the line of the first needle through the stab incision.

Fig. 10.3 Skin markings for arthroscopy.

- The trocar is withdrawn and replaced by the arthroscope.
- The mandible is manipulated by the assistant and the surgeon moves the arthroscope to inspect the upper joint space as continuous irrigation is supplied through the cannula. It is important that the second needle is observed at all times to ensure that flow out of the joint is not impeded.
- A second stab incision may be made about 20 mm in front of, and 5 mm below the first to insert a second cannula. This allows the surgeon to inspect the whole joint from two directions.
- Medicament may be injected, if required, into parts of the joint structure under direct vision.
- The skin is closed at the puncture points with non-absorbable sutures.
- The ear plug is removed.

Post-operative care

- A pressure dressing, if used, is maintained for 24 hours.
- Skin sutures, if non-absorbable, are removed at 5 days.

Complications

- **Haemorrhage:** this is very rare. Pressure should be applied for 15 minutes. It could necessitate an arthrotomy incision to identify the bleeding point.
- **Facial weakness:** if irrigation fluid escapes into the tissues from the joint, pressure on the facial nerve may cause transient facial weakness.
- **Deafness:** this might be due to retention of the ear plug, or blood clot should the ear plug have been displaced during surgery and haemorrhage have been pronounced. The ear should be examined with an auroscope.

Arthroscopic surgery

Recently techniques have been developed using arthroscopy with a further puncture to introduce minute purpose-designed surgical instruments. Lavage can be performed to remove inflammatory substances where synovitis is identified, anti-inflammatory drugs may be injected directly into the inflamed tissues, adhesions incised and procedures on the disc and joint surfaces carried out.

Patient information

This is similar to that for arthroscopy.

Operating theatre procedure

This is identical to that described under arthroscopy. Operating instruments can be inserted through the second cannula according to the surgeon's preferred techniques. This may include diathermy.

Post-operative care and complications

These are also identical to those described under arthroscopy.

Arthrotomy

Aims

As for arthroscopic surgery. Surgery is chiefly in relation to abnormalities and displacement of the disc.

Pre-operative preparation of the patient

- Patient information: this may be in the form of a handout. The operation is through an incision just in front of the ear and running into the hair line. The patient should be warned of possible weakness of the upper part of the face, particularly the forehead and TMJ pain and difficulty in opening the mouth post-operatively.
- Consent.
- Standard check list for general anaesthesia.
- The hair is shaved to remove the sideburn and 2 cm above.

Operating theatre procedure

Instruments required

- 1:100 000 adrenaline solution in saline for skin and joint infiltration
- Instruments for arthrotomy
  - □ Marking pen and Bonney's blue
  - □ Ruler
  - □ Op-site 28 × 30 cm (elliptical hole cut in centre)
  - □ 20 ml syringe with 21G needle
  - □ 1:100 000 adrenaline solution (without local anaesthetic)
  - □ Ear plug (cut from sponge)
  - □ Skin preparation
  - □ Suction tubing, Magill end
  - □ Nos 10 and 15 blades
  - □ Cat's paw retractors
  - □ Self-retaining retractor

- □ 2 × small Langenbeck retractors
- □ Self-retaining Juniper distractor
- □ Drill and No 8 round bur (to prepare bone for distractor)
- □ Sutures according to surgeon's preference
- □ 2 × Howarth periosteal elevator
- □ Mitchells trimmer
- □ Gillies toothed forceps
- □ Fine toothed forceps
- □ Standard needle holder
- □ Fine needle holder
- □ Mayo scissors 6″ curved on flat
- □ Fine scissors curved on flat
- □ Blunt Watson Cheyne
- □ Iris knives
- □ Redivac drain

Anaesthesia

Naso-tracheal intubation with the tube running over the forehead and fixed with adhesive tape. Hypotensive technique may be required.

Position

Standard, with the head supported and turned away from the operating side.

Preparation of the operative site

- ■ Skin preparation
- ■ Standard head towels prepared to expose the side of the face and ear
- ■ Adhesive drape with an oval hole 6 × 4 cm for the pinna
- ■ Plug of plastic foam inserted in the ear

Operative procedure

- ■ The skin is marked and the incision line and tissues posterior to the TMJ are infiltrated with adrenaline solution (Fig. 10.4).

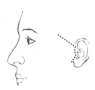

Fig. 10.4 Incision for arthrotomy.

- The incision is taken through the tissues to the zygomatic arch and joint capsule, and raised forward by blunt dissection. A broad periosteal elevator is used.
- Further adrenaline solution is infiltrated into the upper joint space.
- The upper joint space is opened and explored with a blunt instrument and adhesions cut with an iris knife. Most surgeons use a TMJ distractor, and this will require a No 8 round bur on a straight handpiece to prepare for its insertion. The lower joint space is opened and adhesions released as above.
- If a meniscoplasty (meniscopexy) is performed, a wedge will be removed from the back of the meniscus and a 4 mm reverse cutting needle will be used.
- If mobilisation of the meniscus is necessary it is repositioned over the condylar head by carefully placed sutures.
- If a menisectomy is undertaken, the periphery of the meniscus will be cut using a No 15 blade, iris knife and curved scissors. It is essential that no meniscus tissue remains.
- The capsule is closed.
- A vacuum drain is inserted, exiting behind the mastoid process.
- The skin is closed in layers. Many surgeons use a subcuticular suture.
- The ear plug is removed.

Post-operative care

- A pressure dressing, if used, is maintained for 24 hours
- The drain is removed at 24 to 36 hours, after drainage has ceased
- Skin sutures, if non-absorbable, are removed at 7 days

Complications

- **Haemorrhage:** this is rare, but may necessitate removal of some sutures.
- **Facial weakness:** where the joint has not been operated on before, weakness is rare, and then is associated with upper branches of the facial nerve serving the forehead. It is seldom permanent. An untreated haematoma may cause weakness of the whole facial nerve.
- **Deafness:** this is due to either retention of the ear plug or blood clot in the ear. The ear should be examined with an auroscope.
- **Frey syndrome:** inappropriate re-innervation of the sweat glands in the skin over the site of the skin flap by parasympathetic secretomotor nerve fibres from the parotid gland may produce flushing and sweating of the skin with eating – gustatory sweating. This takes months to occur.

Condylectomy

Total condylectomy is performed relatively rarely. Condylar hyperplasia or ankylosis of the TMJ are the most likely reasons. Condylar hyperplasia may result in the mandible on the affected side being thrust downwards or thrust forwards and to the opposite side, so leading to jaw deformity and gross disturbances of the dental occlusion. Ankylosis usually follows infection earlier in life, often from a middle ear infection, which spreads forwards into the TMJ, destroying its architecture and causing fusion between the condyle and the base of the skull. The patient is unable to open the mouth and the mandible does not develop symmetrically, with deviation to the affected side. Bilateral cases can lead to the 'bird face' deformity with the patient appearing to have no chin.

Preparation for the surgery may require extended orthodontic treatment to prepare the dental occlusion for the post-operative corrected position of the mandible.

Pre-operative preparation of the patient

- Patient information: this may be in the form of a handout. The operation is through an incision just in front of the ear and running into the hair line. The patient should be warned of possible weakness of the upper part of the face, particularly the forehead and TMJ pain and difficulty in opening the mouth post-operatively.
- Consent.
- Standard checklist for general anaesthesia.
- The hair is shaved to remove the sideburn and 2 cm above.
- The jaw may deviate to the side of the surgery on mouth opening for some months post-operatively, and will require physiotherapy and home exercises to correct this.

Operating theatre procedure

Instruments required

- Extra-oral soft tissue set
- Drill and saw (*see* Figs 13 and 14)
- 1:100 000 adrenaline solution in saline for skin and joint infiltration

Anaesthesia

Naso-tracheal intubation with the tube running over the forehead and fixed with adhesive tape. Hypotensive technique may be required.

Position

Standard, with the head supported and turned away from the operating side.

Preparation of the operative site

- Skin preparation
- Standard head towels prepared to expose the side of the face and ear
- Adhesive drape with an oval hole 6 × 4 cm for the pinna
- Plug of plastic foam inserted in the ear

Operative procedure

- The skin is marked and the incision line and structures posterior to the TMJ infiltrated with adrenaline solution (*see* Fig. 10.4).
- The incision is taken through the tissues to the zygomatic arch and joint capsule, and raised forward by blunt dissection. A broad periosteal elevator is used.
- The capsule is opened and the condyle is fully exposed as far as the lower part of the condylar neck and, as far as possible, across the top of the condylar head, separating it from the glenoid fossa above. This may be difficult in the case of ankylosis and may require excess bone to be removed with drill, chisel and osteotome.
- The condyle is separated with a drill, saw or osteotome, at the base of the condylar neck in the case of hyperplasia, so as to remove the growth centre and prevent recurrence. In the case of ankylosis, the separation is as low as possible, and may involve a second incision at the angle of the mandible (*see* joint replacement).
- In ankylosis cases some surgeons insert inert foreign material such as silastic, or may advance a temporalis flap into the gap produced. This is to prevent re-ankylosis. The temporalis flap is turned down from the posterior part of the exposure to the joint. Either material is sutured with non-absorbable sutures.
- A vacuum drain is inserted, exiting behind the mastoid process.
- The skin is closed in layers. Many surgeons use a subcuticular suture.
- The ear plug is removed.

Post-operative care

- A pressure dressing, if used, is maintained for 24 hours.
- The drain is removed at 24 to 36 hours after drainage has ceased.
- Skin sutures, if non-absorbable, are removed at 7 days.
- Mouth opening exercises, initially in front of a mirror, are instituted as soon as the patient can tolerate them. In the case of ankylosis, mouth

opening is achieved with a measuring device, such as layered wooden tongue depressors held across the teeth, much as a dog holds a bone, the layers being increased daily until opening of 40 mm or so is achieved and maintained. These exercises are continued for weeks to months.

Complications

- **Haemorrhage:** this is rare, but may necessitate removal of some sutures.
- **Facial weakness:** where the joint has not been operated on before, weakness is rare, and is then associated with upper branches of the facial nerve serving the forehead. It is seldom permanent. An untreated haematoma may cause weakness of the whole facial nerve.
- **Deafness:** this is due to either retention of the ear plug or a blood clot in the ear. The ear should be examined with an auroscope.
- **Frey syndrome:** inappropriate re-innervation of the sweat glands in the skin over the site of the skin flap by parasympathetic secretomotor nerve fibres from the parotid gland may produce flushing and sweating of the skin with eating – gustatory sweating. This takes months to occur.
- The patient may be unable to maintain the gains achieved.

Joint replacement

Aims

To replace the joint with a functional alternative. In the case of a child where continuing growth is required, a costo-chondral graft (the anterior end of a rib) is the most satisfactory. This may be used in the adult where the cartilage of the rib makes a satisfactory joint with the glenoid fossa. Total joint replacements are also available which are made of a combination of metal and plastic. The reason for replacing a joint is following destruction from trauma or disease.

Pre-operative preparation of the patient

- Patient information: this may be in the form of a handout. There will be two incisions, one in front of the ear as described in the operations above, running into the hair line, and a second just beneath the angle of the mandible, about 4 cm long. Both cause potential hazard to the facial nerve, causing weakness of that side of the face. The movement of the forehead muscles and those around the corner of the mouth may be involved. Temporary effects are common, but long-term paralysis rare. There will be pain and difficulty in opening the mouth initially and post-operative exercises will be important.

- Consent.
- Standard checklist for general anaesthesia.
- The hair will be shaved to remove the sideburn and for 2 cm above.

Operating theatre procedure

Instruments required

- Extra-oral soft tissue set
- Drill and saw with irrigation (*see* Figs 4.13 and 4.14)
- Prosthetic joint kit or instruments for taking a rib graft
- 1:100 000 adrenaline solution in saline for skin and joint infiltration

Anaesthesia

Naso-tracheal intubation with the tube running over the forehead and fixed with adhesive tape. Hypotensive technique may be required.

Position

Standard, with the head supported and turned away from the operating side.

Preparation of the operative site

- Skin preparation
- Standard head towels prepared to expose the side of the face and ear, and also the angle of the mandible and point of chin
- Adhesive drape with an oval hole 6 × 4 cm for the pinna
- Plug of plastic foam inserted in the ear

Operative procedure

- The skin is marked and the incision line and tissues posterior to the TMJ are infiltrated with adrenaline solution (*see* Fig. 10.4). A second incision site just below the angle of the mandible is infiltrated too. It is essential that local anaesthetic is not included in the adrenaline solution if a nerve stimulator is to be used as an aid to the identification of the mandibular branch of the facial nerve in the lower incision.
- The pre-auricular incision is taken through the tissues to the zygomatic arch and joint capsule, and raised forward by blunt dissection. A broad periosteal elevator is used.
- The capsule is opened and the condyle is fully exposed as far as the

lower part of the condylar neck and, as far possible, across the top of the condylar head, separating it from the glenoid fossa above.

- A second incision is made at the angle of the mandible. It is designed to run between the mandibular and cervical branches of the facial nerve, and runs for about 4 cm curving around the angle of the mandible.
- The incision is deepened through the skin and fat. As the sub-cutaneous tissues are reached the branches of the facial nerve have to be identified. This is achieved by blunt dissection and most surgeons use a nerve stimulator.
- Once the positions of the branches of the facial nerve have been identified, the incision is deepened to the angle of the mandible from which the periosteum is lifted to meet the dissection from the pre-auricular incision. A tunnel has been created under the facial nerve.
- The condyle is separated with a drill, saw or osteotome. In the case of ankylosis, the separation is as low as possible.
- In ankylosis cases some surgeons insert inert foreign material such as silastic, or may advance a temporalis flap into the gap produced. This is to prevent re-ankylosis. The temporalis flap is turned down from the posterior part of the exposure to the joint. Either material is sutured with non-absorbable sutures.
- Where the joint is being replaced with costo-chondral graft or by a metal prosthesis, the distal ramus is prepared to receive the rib or prosthesis which is fixed by screws or wires.
- A vacuum drain is inserted, exiting behind the mastoid process.
- Both incisions are closed in layers. Many surgeons use a subcuticular suture.
- The ear plug is removed.
- Pressure dressings are applied as required.

Post-operative care

- A pressure dressing, if used, is maintained for 24 hours.
- The drain is removed at 24 to 36 hours after drainage has ceased.
- Skin sutures, if non-absorbable, are removed at 7 days.
- Mouth opening exercises, initially in front of a mirror, are instituted as soon as the patient can tolerate them. In the case of ankylosis, mouth opening is achieved with a measuring device, such layered wooden tongue depressors wedged across the teeth, much as a dog holds a bone, the layers being increased daily until an opening of 40 mm or so is achieved and maintained. These exercises are continued for weeks to months.

Complications

- **Haemorrhage:** this is rare, but may necessitate removal of some sutures.

- **Facial weakness:** where the joint has not been operated on before, weakness is rare, and is then associated with upper branches of the facial nerve serving the forehead. The lower incision lies close to the lower branches of the facial nerve and may lead to weakness of the lower lip. Neither is usually permanent. An untreated haematoma may cause weakness of the whole facial nerve.
- **Deafness:** this is due to either retention of the ear plug or a blood clot in the ear. The ear should be examined with an auroscope.
- **Frey syndrome:** inappropriate re-innervation of the sweat glands in the skin over the site of the skin flap by parasympathetic secretomotor nerve fibres from the parotid gland may produce flushing and sweating of the skin with eating – gustatory sweating. This takes months to occur.
- The patient is unable to maintain the gains achieved.

Dislocation of the TMJ (*see also* Chapter 9)

Acute dislocation

The young female tends to have a laxer joint than the male and an unguarded wide yawn may take the condyle forward of the articular eminence, and muscle spasm of the closing muscles hold it there. It may be very painful and represents an emergency. The sufferer will need hospital treatment in the first instance.

Aims

To reduce the dislocation, if possible, without medication.

Procedure

The operator stands in front of, or behind, the seated patient, with the gloved thumbs wrapped in gauze and placed upon the occlusal surfaces of the mandibular teeth, and the index and middle fingers under the lower border of the mandible. The back of the head should be supported on a head rest – a dental chair is ideal. The mandible is grasped firmly by both hands and a quick thrust is made downwards and backwards, and with a slight rotary movement to bring the condyles back into the fossa (*see* Fig. 9.3). This usually reduces the dislocation. Intravenous sedation may be required, or even a general anaesthetic with muscle relaxant. Thereafter the patient should avoid manoeuvres which cause the jaw to redislocate.

Recurrent dislocation

Recurrent dislocation occurs mainly in two different age groups – the young female and the old and senile. When dislocation is recurrent and the patient becomes a frequent attender at their doctor's surgery or hospital, it is wise to take a psychiatric history as it may be an hysterical or attention-seeking complaint. Where this has been discounted, then operation is indicated. The elderly and senile may dislocate recurrently for entirely different reasons, for example incoordination of the jaw muscles, maybe as a result of previous phenothiazine therapy. Surgery may be the only recourse.

The operations fall into two groups, but both are directed to the articular eminence. The eminence can either be enhanced to prevent forward translation and dislocation of the mandible or removed (eminectomy) so that the dislocated condyle may slide back uninhibited. All the devised operations have their proponents and detractors and none are guaranteed successful unless the patient can co-operate in avoiding very wide mouth opening post-operatively.

Pre-operative preparation of the patient

- Patient information: this may be in the form of a handout. The operation is through an incision just in front of the ear and running into the hair line. The patient should be warned of possible weakness of the upper part of the face, particularly the forehead, and TMJ pain and difficulty in opening the mouth post-operatively.
- Consent.
- Standard checklist for general anaesthesia.
- The hair is shaved to remove the sideburn and 2 cm above.

Operating theatre procedure

Instruments required

- Extra-oral soft tissue set
- Drill and saw with irrigation (*see* Figs 13 and 14)
- 1:100 000 adrenaline solution in saline for skin and joint infiltration

Anaesthesia

Naso-tracheal intubation with the tube running over the forehead and fixed with adhesive tape.

Position

Standard, with the head supported and turned away from the operating side.

Preparation of the operative site

■ Skin preparation
■ Standard head towels prepared to expose the side of the face and ear
■ Adhesive drape with an oval hole 6 × 4 cm for the pinna
■ Plug of plastic foam inserted in the ear

Operative procedure

■ The skin is marked and the pre-auricular incision line is infiltrated with adrenaline solution.
■ The incision is taken through the tissues to the zygomatic arch and joint capsule, and raised forward by blunt dissection. A broad periosteal elevator is used.
■ The eminence and zygomatic arch are exposed, but the joint capsule is not opened.
■ If an eminectomy is performed, a bur or osteotome is placed at the root of the eminence at right angles to the arch, and the eminence is simply separated off the bone above. The resulting bony platform is smoothed and flattened.
■ If the eminence is to be increased, suitable bone has to be harvested from another site – the point of the chin is the most accessible and has the least morbidity. This is done by an intra-oral approach. It may then be attached directly to the eminence by a bone screw or wedged into the existing eminence which is split obliquely from the posterior aspect and downfractured.

A further variant of eminence augmentation is achieved by an operation whereby the root of the zygoma is separated obliquely from the eminence and sprung medially and downward to lie below the eminence. It may be left free or fixed with a wire or screw.

All these augmentation operations may fail where the condyle is small, as it may slip by the augmented eminence on its medial side when the mouth opens.

■ A vacuum drain may be inserted, exiting behind the mastoid process.
■ The incision is closed in layers. Many surgeons use a subcuticular suture.
■ The ear plug is removed.
■ Pressure dressings are applied as required.

Post-operative care

■ A pressure dressing, if used, is maintained for 24 hours.
■ The drain, if used, is removed at 24 to 36 hours after drainage has ceased.

- Skin sutures, if non-absorbable, are removed at 7 days.
- Mouth opening is discouraged. (Some surgeons use intermaxillary fixation for 10 days.)

Complications

- **Haemorrhage:** this is rare, but may necessitate removal of some sutures.
- **Facial weakness:** this is rare, and is then associated with upper branches of the facial nerve serving the forehead. It is seldom permanent.
- **Deafness:** this is due to either retention of the ear plug or a blood clot in the ear. The ear should be examined with an auroscope.
- **Frey syndrome:** inappropriate re-innervation of the sweat glands in the skin over the site of the skin flap by parasympathetic secretomotor nerve fibres from the parotid gland may produce flushing and sweating of the skin with eating – gustatory sweating. This takes months to occur.
- The patient may dislocate again.

Summary

Facial arthromyalgia (TMJ dysfunction) is a common disorder which is treated conservatively in the out-patient clinic. Surgical conditions are less common, but treatment may involve major operative procedures and prolonged rehabilitation.

11

Part I
Malignancy of the Maxillofacial Region

P.J. Leopard

This chapter describes the presentation and treatment of cancer in the maxillofacial area. The epidemiology and aetiology are outlined as well as the diagnoses. The rationale for treatment and different treatment modalities are discussed. Examples are given of surgery at specific sites. Appropriate after care is covered including the role of the head and neck nurse specialist.

Epidemiology and aetiology

Despite advances in the diagnosis and management in the past 40 years the cure rate of most oral cancers has not improved significantly. In the United Kingdom there are around 2000 new cases of cancer of the lip, tongue and oral cavity each year and around 1000 deaths from the disease. It is the eighth commonest cancer in developed countries and the third commonest in developing countries. In some parts of India it is the commonest of all cancers, comprising 40% of all malignant disease compared to 1% of all cancers in the UK, a similar incidence to cancer of the cervix.

Although 85% of cases occur in people aged over 50 years and twice as many cases occur in men than in women, recent trends are significantly towards a younger age group in both sexes.

Risk factors include a positive family history, dietary deficiency (vitamins A, C and iron) but most significantly of all the use of tobacco and alcohol. Those who smoke over 20 cigarettes a day are 10 times more likely to develop oral cancer than non-smokers; those who drink over six ounces (180 ml) of alcohol a day are 2.5 times more likely to develop oral cancer than tee-totallers. Those who do both increase the risk by a striking factor of 24. Primary preventive measures are obvious and should be promoted by the maxillofacial team. Secondary preventive measures should be directed towards early diagnosis. Patients diagnosed early have significantly better survival rates and require less radical treatment. Delays in patient presentation, referral by general practitioners, and the recognition and treatment of certain pre-cancerous conditions can all be addressed by raising public awareness and the education of general practitioners respectively. Screening programmes other than regular oral inspections for all are of benefit only to the high-risk groups.

Presentation

Oral cancer

Most oral cancers present as irregular craggy ulcers with raised edges, often within a surrounding area of thickened leukoplakia. They are frequently painless and therefore may have reached a considerable size. As the tumour enlarges there may be difficulty with speech and swallowing, an unpleasant odour and drooling. Early cancers may appear as shallow erosions, as papilliferous growths or as hard swellings below the surface.

Sinus cancer

Cancer of the maxillary sinus may appear as a facial swelling or as a swelling of the upper alveolus or within the nose. There may be facial numbness, nasal obstruction with or without bleeding or, if the tumour has spread into the orbit, the globe of the eye may be displaced with accompanying double vision (diplopia).

Skin cancer

See Chapter 11, Part II.

Classification and staging

Tumours of the head and neck may by classified according to their type and location and staged according to their degree of local, regional and distant spread. Typically, most primary cancers of the oro-facial region spread by local invasion initially, somewhat later by spread to the regional lymph nodes and much later by distant spread (metastasis) via the blood stream to other parts of the body. It is not uncommon for some patients with oral cancer to have a second cancer elsewhere in the aero-digestive tract (mouth, pharynx, larynx and bronchus). Different histo-logical cancers have different behaviour patterns in this respect, some being much more aggressive than others. Thus, it is important to classify and stage every cancer so that the best treatment protocol can be chosen and so some idea of prognosis given.

Classification

There are four main groups of cancer in the oro-facial region:

- Squamous carcinoma of the mucosal surfaces of the mouth, sinuses, pharynx and larynx
- Basal cell and squamous cell carcinomas and melanomas of the facial skin
- Tumours of the salivary glands (*see* Chapter 8)
- Lymphomas

Other cancers include rare secondary deposits from elsewhere.

Apart from skin cancers, the relative incidence of the remainder is:

- Mucosal squamous carcinoma – 75.0%
- Salivary tumours – 7.5%
- Lymphomas – 2.5%
- Miscellaneous – 15.0%

Staging

Staging of oral cancer is by the TNM system (the size and other features of the primary **T**umour, the presence and location of the regional lymph **N**odes and the presence of distant **M**etastases – *see* Table 11.1).

Table 11.1   TNM staging

Tumour	T0	No evidence of primary tumour
	T$_{IS}$	Pre-invasive (carcinoma *in situ*)
	T1	Up to 2 cm diameter
	T2	2–4 cm diameter
	T3	Over 4 cm diameter
	T4	Deep invasion with bone/muscle/skin involvement
Nodes	N0	No clinical nodes
	N1	Ipsilateral node <3 cm
	N2	Bilateral or contralateral nodes <6 cm
	N3	Node(s) >6 cm
Metastases	M0	No distant spread
	M1	Evidence of distant spread

Diagnosis

All suspected malignant lesions must be biopsied. There are three principal types of biopsy:

- **Incisional biopsy**, where a segment of tissue is taken from the margin of the lesion to include its edge and a portion of adjacent normal tissue.
- **Excisional biopsy**, where for a small lesion it is excised completely with an appropriate normal margin.
- **Fine needle aspiration (FNA) cytology**, where cells from a suspected tumour deep to the surface are 'sucked out' and transferred to make a smear on a glass slide.

Incisional biopsy is the method of choice for all surface lesions of the mucous membranes and skin suspected of malignancy. Excisional biopsy is used for small benign lesions. Where the subsequent histological report demonstrates an unsuspected malignancy the surgeon must decide between continuing close observation or a more radical definitive operation to ensure that a wider clear margin has been achieved. Fine needle aspiration is used chiefly for the diagnosis of parotid tumours (*see* Chapter 8) and to determine whether lymph node enlargement is due to malignant involvement or inflammatory changes. Biopsies are usually carried out in the out-patient setting under local anaesthesia.

Biopsy techniques (*see also* Chapter 6)

Incisional biopsy

Requirements:

- Local anaesthetic
- Standard set for intra-oral biopsy/soft tissue surgery (*see* Fig. 4.7)
- Specimen pot(s) with formol saline
- Histopathology request forms

Local regional or field anaesthesia is used to avoid injecting into the lesion and distorting its histological appearance or the theoretical risk of spreading malignant cells. The specimen is placed immediately into formol saline (formalin) and dispatched with the appropriate histopathology request form. The wound is sutured with resorbable or non-resorbable sutures.

If multiple biopsies are taken it is important that the surgeon identifies the site of each and that they are clearly distinguished in separate specimen bottles. The same technique is used for specimens taken for immediate frozen section during operations, to establish margins of clearance or involvement of lymph nodes, except that the specimen is not placed in formalin.

Excisional biopsy

The technique is identical, but the specimen comprises the entire visible lesion. The somewhat larger defect is closed by undermining the wound edges to allow primary suture or by the rotation of a small local flap of mucosa or skin.

FNA cytology

Requirements:

- Standard 10 to 20 ml plastic syringe
- Standard disposable needle (22 to 25 g)
- Clean dry glass microscope slides/cover slips
- Fixing agent – alcohol or hairspray

The cytopathologist or laboratory assistant is usually present to prepare the slide and transport it immediately to the laboratory.

The needle is attached to the syringe and then advanced vertically into the centre of the lump concerned. Local anaesthesia is usually not required. When in position, the plunger is drawn back to create a vacuum which is maintained whilst the assembled syringe and needle are moved backwards and forwards and in different directions. The effect within the tumour is that the sharp bevelled edge of the needle harvests cells, which are drawn back into the lumen of the needle. Unless the mass contains fluid, nothing appears within the syringe.

When the movements are complete, the suction is released and the syringe and needle withdrawn. The needle is then disconnected, air drawn into the syringe, the needle reconnected and the specimen expelled as a single drop onto clean glass slides. The edge of a slide or cover slip then is used to drag the contents of the drop into a smear. This dries in air rapidly. The cytologist usually determines whether the specimen should be fixed using alcohol or even hair spray before transporting it to the laboratory.

Other diagnostic procedures

Imaging

Standard plain films are taken (usually an OPT and/or sinus views) in all cases to determine any gross bone involvement and the presence of other pathology such as retained or infected dental roots.

MRI or CT scans are necessary to determine the extent of local spread and the involvement of lymph nodes. Unfortunately, even the most sophisticated techniques are unable to pick up very small nodes or early bone involvement but are, nevertheless, extremely useful. Occasionally other imaging techniques such as angiography, radionucleotide imaging and ultrasound are indicated in specific circumstances.

A chest X-ray is mandatory to determine the presence of any distant metastases or other significant cardiorespiratory disease.

Haematological and biochemical tests

Patients with oral cancer may have a dietary deficiency and all those requiring surgery will require blood tests. These tests will include a full blood count and ESR, coagulation screening, grouping and later cross-matching of blood, and a range of serum biochemistry which may include estimations of iron, vitamins C and B12, folate, liver, cardiac and bone enzymes in addition to urea and electrolytes as tests of renal function.

Endoscopy

The use of flexible fibre-optic endoscopes is standard practice in the out-patient setting and enables a thorough examination of the nose, naso-pharynx, hypopharynx and glottis to determine the presence of other lesions and the extent of a posterior oral lesion beyond the visible area.

The procedure of endoscopy may be carried out under local (topical) anaesthesia with or without intravenous sedation, or under general anaesthesia prior to making a decision to operate.

Endoscopes are expensive instruments and training in their care and maintenance is necessary. They require a light source and have a variety of biopsy forceps, curettes and suction tips. Their optical properties depend on factors such as their diameter and the type and angulation of the lens at their navigable tip. This ability to see and operate round corners enables the surgeon to plan the extent of ablative surgery or even to decide that a tumour is too extensive and thus inoperable.

Multidisciplinary clinics

Patients with cancer of the maxillofacial region must be assessed and have their treatment planned in joint, multidisciplinary clinics, which should also be the setting for their continued follow-up and where record keeping, audit and research can be standardised and coordinated. In any centre treating an adequate number of such patients, these clinics should be held weekly or, at the most, fortnightly and a designated liaison nurse should be available and known to the patients at all times (*see* Chapter 11, part III).

The full team will comprise maxillofacial, ENT (ear, nose and throat) and plastic surgeons, radiotherapists/oncologists, histopathologist, link or liaison nurse, speech therapist, dietician, restorative dentist, hygienist, clinical photographer and maxillofacial technician along with trainees in these areas of expertise. Clearly, to assemble this group in one room is neither possible nor desirable. The system should be organised so that the essential clinicians and nurses are present and that those less central to immediate decisions are readily available on site.

Patients and their relatives must be afforded sensitivity, courtesy and dignity in calm surroundings. Breaking bad news is a skill, which must allow time for the reaction of the patients and family to take place in privacy but without a feeling of isolation. The maxillofacial nurse has a key role to play in this context and will be able to offer reassurance, a full explanation of the treatment that lies ahead, counselling, links with patient groups, pain relief services and, when necessary, hospice and terminal care introduction. Patients may need dietary advice, prosthetic help and a wide variety of support services at any time and must know to whom they can turn at any time.

Treatment

Once the diagnosis has been made and the treatment options considered in full consultation with the patient, a clear treatment plan with objectives is agreed. The objectives are most commonly to try to eradicate the disease and rehabilitate the patient to as normal a life as possible. However, in advanced disease or sometimes in deference to a patient's wishes, the aim is to contain the disease as well as possible and for as long as possible with a minimum of suffering. Thus, the choice is to aim for a cure or to palliate and in either case to best preserve the quality of life. The results of treatment must never be worse than the disease itself.

The three main treatment modalities are:

- Surgical excision
- Radiotherapy
- Chemotherapy

Combinations of the above are frequently used.

Surgery

With modern techniques and anaesthesia, almost all head and neck tumours can be surgically removed. However, bearing in mind the need also to resect a wide three-dimensional margin of normal tissue, such surgery can be debilitating if not mutilating and may not be the treatment of choice. Other factors such as the patient's extreme age, other physical debility and the presence of inoperable neck nodes or distant metastases may mitigate against surgery as the primary treatment of choice.

In the presence of incurable disease, surgery may be palliative to improve the quality of remaining life. Where surgery is selected to attempt a cure, the following principles must be followed:

- The entire tumour must be removed. This should include a reasonable margin of surrounding normal tissue as well as involved regional lymph nodes and the intervening tissue.
- Every attempt should be made to reconstruct the defect to reproduce form and function as completely as possible. A range of highly successful reconstructive procedures is available.

Where there is conflict between these principles, the adequacy of resection should not be compromised. It is better to accept some deformity or disability than to remove a tumour incompletely.

Radiotherapy

Radiotherapy may be curative or palliative. It is delivered either by external beam or by brachytherapy – the insertion of radioactive implants within the tumour, to a prescription ordered by the radiotherapist and calculated by the medical physicist.

Within a few weeks of being irradiated, all tissues begin to undergo permanent changes which adversely affect surgical healing and it is rarely possible to repeat radiotherapy at the same site. Other changes such as early mucositis within the mouth and severe desquamation of the facial skin recover to a large extent once treatment has finished. Serious wound breakdown is a likely consequence of surgery performed after radiotherapy. Nowhere is this more so than in bone.

Radiotherapy can permanently affect the salivary and mucous glands, giving rise to permanent dryness of the mouth leading to a sharp increase in dental caries and susceptibility to candidal infection as well as difficulty with speech and swallowing due to poor lubrication. Traditionally, external beam radiotherapy is delivered over 6 or 7 weeks, patients attending for treatment several days a week. Treatment is sometimes accelerated using two or three fractions a day, the course being completed much more rapidly.

Chemotherapy

Apart from the lymphomas and in late palliation, chemotherapy is rarely, if ever, used as the primary treatment of choice in head and neck cancer. All drugs used in chemotherapy have a high toxicity, particularly affecting the bone marrow, kidneys, ears, hair and gastro-intestinal system. Various combinations of drugs have been used over the years directed in the UK by the UK Co-ordinating Committee for Cancer Research. Early encouraging response rates to drugs such as methotrexate, cisplatin and fluorouracil have not been sustained. These agents are now used synchronously with radiotherapy or for palliating very extensive disease.

Factors influencing the choice of treatment

Although for relatively small tumours, surgery and radiotherapy are equally successful, radiotherapy may give better functional results. Very extensive tumours, especially towards the pharynx, may be inoperable and better treated by radiotherapy. Carcinoma of the nasopharynx and early cancer of the larynx respond very well to radiotherapy. However, if a tumour recurs after radiotherapy, surgical cure is much less likely. In addition, tumours involving bone, multifocal tumours and those with involved regional lymph nodes are better treated surgically. Very large tumours do not respond well to radiotherapy because of their bulk (volume) and unless the aim is palliation, are better dealt with by surgery. Where the regional lymph nodes are involved, these and the primary tumour are removed surgically. If the subsequent histological examination demonstrates extracapsular spread of cells outside the lymph node, or where there is inadequate clearance of the primary tumour, post-operative radiotherapy is given.

There is much debate concerning the management of the neck without clinically involved nodes. Undoubtedly a significant number of these patients later develop nodal disease. Some surgeons believe that a modified radical neck dissection should be carried out even when there are no clinically obvious nodes when the primary tumour is treated surgically, and that the neck should also be included in the field when the primary tumour is treated by radiotherapy.

Surgery at specific sites

Lower lip

Following resection of the tumour, the lower lip may be reconstructed by direct closure of a central defect or by a rotation flap such as the fan flap if the defect is close to the corner of the mouth (Fig. 11.1(a) and (b)).

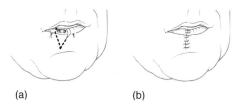

(a)   (b)

Fig. 11.1(a) and (b)   Direct closure of lower lip following wedge excision.

Anterior floor of the mouth

Many smaller carcinomas of the anterior floor of mouth can be excised intra-orally. Those that involve the alveolar mucosa or the body of the tongue require an approach similar to that described later for the posterior floor of mouth. A clear margin of at least 1 cm should be included, which invariably involves the submandibular ducts.

Repair is by the use of one or two nasolabial flaps (Fig. 11.2(a) and (b)) or by free tissue transfer using the radial forearm flap (*see below*).

Anterior tongue

Smaller (T1 or T2) carcinomas of the anterior free part of the tongue without involved lymph nodes can be treated by surgical excision or by radiotherapy. Where lymph nodes are involved, treatment is by *en bloc* removal of the primary tumour and lymph nodes in continuity. This can sometimes be accomplished by a 'pull through' procedure, but is usually best managed by dividing the lip and mandible to enable better access for resection and reconstruction. Partial glossectomy for small tumours is

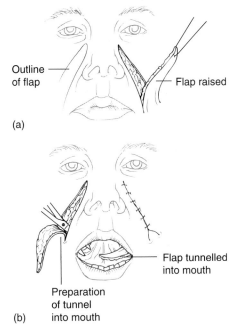

Outline of flap — Flap raised

(a)

Flap tunnelled into mouth

Preparation of tunnel into mouth

(b)

Fig. 11.2(a) and (b) The use of nasolabial flaps tunnelled in through the cheek to repair a floor of mouth defect.

followed by a split skin graft or merely by allowing the area to heal spontaneously. Although functional results for this type of tumour are probably better following radiotherapy, the anterior tongue adapts extremely well to partial loss of substance.

Posterior tongue, floor of mouth and retromolar region

Posterior tumours of the oral cavity tend to be noticed later by patients and are usually more advanced at presentation both in terms of their size and the likelihood of lymph node involvement. By the same criteria they are more likely to have invaded adjacent muscle and bone. Treatment is therefore more radical and involves wide local resection, often including a significant length of mandibular bone, some form of neck dissection and careful reconstruction of bone and oral soft tissues, as well as overlying skin if that has been involved.

These can be very lengthy procedures and, throughout the procedure, the patient must be kept warm and due attention paid to blood loss and fluid balance. At the outset arterial and venous lines are inserted and a urinary catheter placed. A tracheostomy is performed if post operative airway problems are envisaged.

The resection

Skin markings are drawn to indicate the incisions and anatomical landmarks. It is helpful to tattoo a series of dots each side of incisions using a needle with Bonney's blue or toluidine blue dye to aid accurate closure.

Skin and mucosal flaps are raised. Access to the tumour is greatly facilitated by division of the lower lip and the mandible anterior to the mental nerve. The lower face may then be swung laterally to give a clear view of the area to be removed (Fig. 11.3). A cutting diathermy is used to restrict blood loss and to reduce the theoretical chance of shed malignant cells entering blood vessels. Where bone is to be removed, so is the overlying periosteum. Bone is divided using a powered saw. Before the cuts are completed, it is helpful to fashion a titanium reconstruction plate and to drill the screw holes so that the fragments either side of the gap can be accurately repositioned during reconstruction.

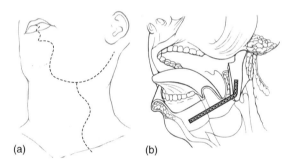

(a)   (b)

Fig. 11.3(a) and (b)   Illustrates how division of the lower lip assists access and showing the use of a reconstruction plate following mandibular resection.

The neck dissection

The objective is to remove all regional lymph nodes that may be involved. They are arranged anatomically in five levels from the lower border of the mandible down to the posterior triangle of the neck above the outer end of the clavicle (Fig. 11.4).

Various types of neck dissection are performed, from the radical neck dissection which includes all the lymph nodes, the sternomastoid muscle, the internal jugular vein and the accessory nerve, to various types of modified radical neck dissection which spare one or more of the latter three structures. Selective dissections are sometimes performed leaving one or more of the five groups of lymph nodes.

Various skin incisions are available, the choice depending on operator preference, the desirability not to have a suture line directly over the carotid vessels and whether a bulky muscle pedicle is to be located under the skin flap (Fig. 11.5(a) and (b)).

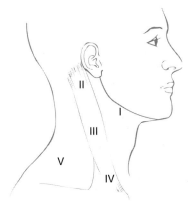

Fig. 11.4 The five levels at which lymph nodes may be involved.

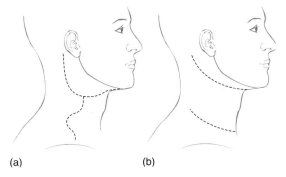

Fig. 11.5 Two commonly used incisions for neck dissection, the 'Y' incision (a) and the McFee (b).

The reconstruction

The need to restore form and function has generated the development of a huge variety of reconstructive techniques. In the maxillofacial region these may be grouped as follows:

Free tissue transfer
This involves the harvesting of tissue – skin, fascia and/or adjacent bone – from a distant site together with the arteries and veins that supply it, transferring that composite structure and joining (anastamosing) its blood vessels to those near the defect so that the transferred tissue immediately takes on an adequate blood supply. The anastamoses are usually performed under the operating microscope, but magnifying loupes may also be used. There is a range of delicate expensive instruments and sutures dedicated to microvascular work, which must never be used for other purposes (*see* microsurgical instrument section in Chapter 4).

Common examples of the donor sites used in free tissue transfer are:

- Radial forearm   – skin and fascia (may include radial bone)
- Latissimus dorsi – muscle and skin
- Rectus abdominis – muscle and skin
- Scapular   – skin (may include bone)
- Fibular   – bone and skin
- Iliac (DCIA)   – bone of pelvic rim
- Rib   – bone

Each has advantages and disadvantages, particularly in relation to the length of the vascular pedicle. The commonest used in the maxillofacial region is the radial forearm flap (Fig. 11.6). The skin it provides is relatively thin and pliable. The donor site is usually closed with either a split skin graft or a full thickness graft of abdominal skin.

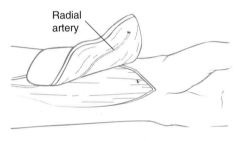

Fig. 11.6   Raising the radial forearm flap.

Axial flaps
Developed before free tissue transfer, axial flaps are islands of tissue which remain attached to their major blood supply and which are mobilised and relocated to a surgical defect. Two examples still in common use are:

- Pectoralis major   – muscle and skin (Fig. 11.7)
- Temporalis   – muscle (sometimes cranial bone) (Fig. 11.8)

These flaps tend to be used where there is a need for bulk, where a free flap has failed or where the operating time or facilities are restricted.

Random flaps
These rely on adjacent tissue for their blood supply. Fortunately this is very adequate in the maxillofacial region. Many examples are given in Chapter 11, Part II, in the section on skin cancer, but two examples used for oral reconstruction are:

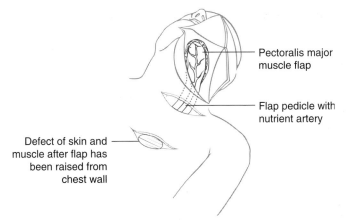

Fig. 11.7   Raising the pectoralis major flap from the chest wall. The nutrient vessels can be seen on the deep surface of the flap which is tunnelled under the skin of the neck to reach the mouth.

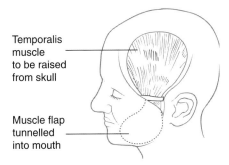

Fig. 11.8   The temporalis flap comprising muscle and overlying fascia is passed through the pterygoid region to reach the oral cavity.

- Naso-labial flaps (*see* Fig. 11.2(a) and (b))
- Tongue flaps

Restoration of bone defect
Where a mandibular defect is created, this may be reconstructed by means of a composite free flap containing bone (fibula, rib, iliac crest, split radius and cranial bone) or a heavy-duty titanium reconstruction plate. If bone is used, osseointegrated implants can be considered later (*see* Chapter 12). Posterior bony defects of the mandible need not be reconstructed.

During lengthy ablative and reconstructive surgery, it is usual for the neck dissection to be carried out early on. The surgeons then split into two teams, one continuing with the resection, the other raising and preparing the reconstructive flap. After resection of the tumour, frozen sections are often taken to make sure that all malignant tissue has been removed. The results are usually transmitted by telephone within 30 minutes. The teams then join together for the lengthy process of suturing the flaps into place and closing the skin.

The resected specimen should be 'pegged out' on a cork board and labelled so that the histopathologist can comment on particular areas. When 'pegged out' the specimen and board are placed in a suitable container of formalin.

Maxillary sinus

Carcinoma of the antrum is treated by the operation of maxillectomy. For small lesions situated low and anterior, this may be carried out through the mouth. For larger tumours it is necessary to divide the upper lip and swing the mid-facial skin laterally to get access to the upper and posterior parts of the maxilla (Fig. 11.9(a) and (b)). If the floor of the orbit is involved by tumour, an exenteration of the entire orbital contents is necessary. It is essential to repair the maxillary defect immediately, usually with a pre-constructed obturator and sometimes by a flap. Obturators are constructed by the maxillofacial technician, and used to carry a split skin graft which will line the maxillectomy cavity. The immediate (operative) obturator, constructed of acrylic (plastic) and gutta percha or lightweight foam, remains in position for several weeks. After the initial healing phase, a permanent obturator is made. This is a removable appliance and its construction is a lengthy clinical and laboratory process, but is carried out on an out-patient basis. Patients with maxillary defects experience major problems with speech and swallowing unless an obturator is fitted. During the early weeks the obturator must not be left out for more then 30 minutes, as the cavity can close down rapidly and prevent re-insertion. Patients will need instruction in the

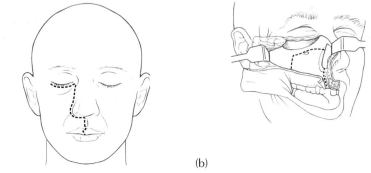

(a)   (b)

Fig. 11.9 Facial incisions (a) and bony cuts (b) for a hemimaxillectomy. (Intra-oral bony cuts are also required.)

insertion, removal and care of their obturator as well as the care of the maxillectomy cavity.

Post-operative care

Patients undergoing major maxillofacial surgery are usually transferred directly from the operating theatre to the intensive care/therapy unit (ITU), where a range of requirements can be met.

Airway management

Because of anticipated local swelling, patients will leave the operating theatre with a tracheostomy tube or nasotracheal tube in place and mechanical ventilation continued in the ITU. Detailed consideration of airway management in the ITU is beyond the scope of this book but failure of oxygenation may be due to a number of causes such as areas of collapse of lung tissue, airway obstruction or the persisting effects of anaesthetic agents. Humidified air with an oxygen concentration of 40% is used.

A chest X-ray may be required to identify collapse or pneumothorax. Steroids are prescribed to reduce post-operative swelling.

Pain relief

In the early post-operative period morphine or pethidine is usually given by infusion. Later, patients may control their own dosage with either a subcutaneous or intravenous patient controlled administration system (PCA). Non-steroidal anti-inflammatory drugs such as diclofenac sodium are useful and may be given per rectum.

Anticoagulation

Heparin-controlled anticoagulation is frequently used to prevent coagulation at the site of the vascular anastamosis and reduce the risk of deep vein thrombosis. The use of heparin carries the risk of post-operative bleeding and is therefore not prolonged. Low dose subcutaneous heparin and the use of TED stockings until the patient is mobile are standard practice.

Hypothermia

Lowering of the body temperature during long operations may be due to the operative transfusion of blood or other fluids that are too cool or to loss of body heat due to exposure. These are preventable by using a warming mattress and only transfusing fluids at body heat. Shivering in the post-operative period is undesirable and may be due to heat loss.

Fluid balance

Operative blood loss, pre-operative fasting and inadequate fluid replacement can all lead to a significant deficit of fluid volume. Fluid balance is monitored by measuring urinary output, central venous pressure, arterial pressure and heart rate. This is a most important feature of post-operative nursing care.

Nutrition

Clearly, swallowing may be seriously affected by major maxillofacial surgery, yet a balanced nutrition is essential for normal healing. In the short term this may be accomplished by intravenous feeding (total parenteral nutrition or TPN) or via a nasogastric tube. Neither is satisfactory for lengthy periods and PEG (percutaneous endoscopic gastrostomy) feeding via a tube inserted through the abdominal wall into the stomach may be required.

Summary

Given the special nature of its site, oral cancer even if successfully treated, may have a devastating effect on a patient's life. Modern techniques have improved the quality of life for many patients, but most will require considerable support following treatment. The emphasis throughout management is on multidisciplinary teamwork, and on early diagnosis brought about by increasing public awareness of the condition with easy access to diagnostic expertise.

11

Part II
Skin Cancer

M. Telfer

This section contains a description of the presentation and treatment of skin cancers of the facial area. In contrast to the prognosis for cancer arising from the skin of the mouth (mucous membrane) the prognosis for cancer of the skin of the face and scalp is excellent. Treatment is primarily surgical and a wide range of techniques for excision and repair is described together with details of postoperative wound care.

Skin cancers

This group of cancers comprises:

- Basal cell carcinoma (rodent ulcer)
- Squamous cell carcinoma
- Melanoma

Basal cell carcinoma (BCC) (Fig. 11.10)

The skin of the head and neck region is the site for 80–85% of all basal cell carcinomas (BCCs), the most frequent skin cancer, which is hardly surprising as the common epidermal tumours are all related to cumulative exposure to ultraviolet light. The BCC is often known as a rodent ulcer because of its slow progressive enlargement and central ulceration, but the presentation is varied and may simply be classified as:

- Nodular
- Ulcerative
- Morphoeic (sclerotic)
- Cystic
- Pigmented

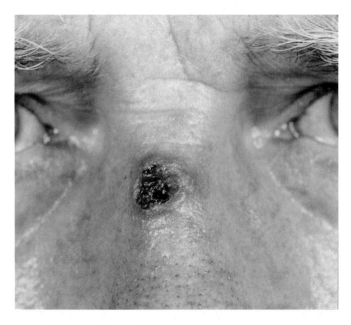

Fig. 11.10   Basal cell carcinoma of the nose.

Clinically it is better to divide them into tumours with or without a clearly defined edge, that is localised or infiltrating, and surgical excision must take this into account. These skin cancers are slow growing and do not metastasise but cause local damage, especially if neglected (Fig. 11.11).

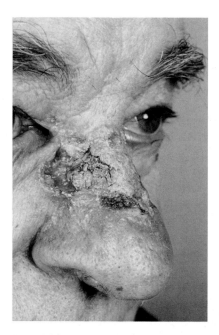

Fig. 11.11 Neglected basal cell carcinoma of the nose.

Squamous cell carcinoma (SCC)

This arises in sun-damaged skin, especially of the scalp and ear, presenting as a raised nodule, an ulcer with raised everted edge or as a fungating fleshy lesion (Fig. 11.12). Differentiation between SCC and BCC is sometimes difficult, but with SCC metastasis to the lymph nodes of the neck may occur, and their rate of growth is greater.

Kerato acanthoma (KA) is a rapidly developing, but benign and self-limiting tumour which presents as a dome shaped lesion with a central keratotic core, often with vertical sides. Because it is often difficult to differentiate clinically and histologically between KA and SCC, excision is frequently recommended if regression is not apparent within a few months.

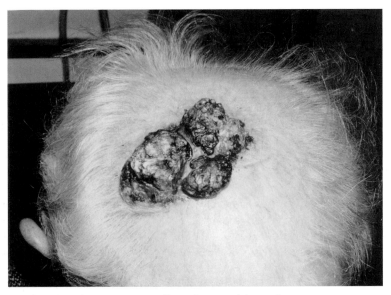

Fig. 11.12   Fungating squamous cell carcinoma of the scalp.

Melanoma

The incidence of this more serious skin cancer is doubling each decade in the United Kingdom with it affecting a younger age range and carrying an overall mortality of 40 to 45%. Although more common elsewhere on the body (men – back, women – leg), it may be seen on the skin of the head and neck. Lentigo maligna is a pigmented patch on the face which slowly enlarges, shows atypia of the melanocytes histologically and has the potential to develop into lentigo maligna melanoma. Early surgical excision is increasingly advised.

Melanoma is classified as follows:

- Superficial spreading melanoma   – the commonest type
- Nodular melanoma   – the most aggressive type
- Lentigo maligna melanoma   – the type most likely to affect the face of the elderly

- Acral or acral-lentiginous melanoma

Diagnosis

Diagnosis of all skin tumours is by clinical recognition, biopsy (*see* Chapters 6 and 11, Part I) or a combination. Incision or punch biopsies take a small representative portion of the tumour with or without normal skin, to establish diagnosis before definitive treatment. Small lesions may be dealt with by excision biopsy if primary closure is simple.

Management

Surgical excision and reconstruction is the treatment of choice in the majority of skin cancers, although radiotherapy is equally effective in mid range 1 to 2 cm tumours, but is best avoided in younger patients and is poorly tolerated in severely sun-damaged skin.

- **Basal cell carcinomas** are excised with a margin of 5 mm, but those with poorly defined margins are more difficult to assess and require excision in experienced units. The use of multiple frozen sections or Moh's micrographic surgery, can be useful in certain anatomical sites to determine clearance whilst minimising damage. Moh's surgery involves excision with chemical cauterisation and multiple repeated biopsies, until the margins are tumour free. Popular in the USA, it is time consuming and costly but offers advantages in the ill defined morphoeic BCC type especially in the nasal and eye regions.
- **Squamous cell carcinomas and melanomas** are excised slightly more widely. The margin of excision for melanomas has decreased over the years as prospective trials have shown no disadvantage in outcome with smaller margins, and now current guidelines indicate margins of 1 to 3 cm, depending on the depth and size of the melanoma.

Excision of all skin cancers involves the deeper tissues as well as peripheral skin and this is of great significance in the head and neck region. Deep excision on the trunk or leg is straightforward as the subcutaneous layer of fat is considerable and allows excision margins to be easily achieved without involving important nearby vessels or structures. This is not the case on the face, scalp or neck where margins of excision are affected by the close proximity of vital structures, for example eye, facial nerve, nasal cartilages, or by the limited depth of tissues available for excision such as on the scalp. Achieving an adequate margin of clearance around and beneath the tumour on the face may often involve compromise to preserve important structures and minimise aesthetic damage. The design of the excision to facilitate the best functional and aesthetic reconstruction of the facial defect is of great importance to the individual patient. The skill is in achieving surgical excision of the tumour while minimising the damage.

Reconstruction of cutaneous surgical defects involves a choice depending on several factors and takes into consideration the defect, the patient and the complexity of reconstructive techniques available. A particular reconstructive technique may offer a clearly superior result, but if not, the simplest choice is usually the best choice.

Reconstructive options

- No repair   – healing by secondary intention
- Primary repair – low tension primary closure
- Skin graft   – split or full thickness skin or composite graft
- Local flap

No repair

Small defects in concave areas can heal with good functional and aesthetic results, and this technique may be useful in larger areas in some patients where contraction of the wound during healing is not important. Longer healing time, increased wound care and poorer cosmesis must be taken into account.

Wound care post-operatively

- Non-adherent dressing applied to wound
- Tie-over packs often used and removed at 7 to 10 days
- Aseptic removal of dressing and sutures
- Wound may be left exposed and daily cleaning at home with sterile saline or boiled water
- Application of Polyfax antibiotic ointment to exposed wound

Primary repair

This is simple, quick and satisfactory if skin tension is low at closure; the final scar will lie in a favourable skin line and no dog ears result. Long suture lines should be avoided as these scars are easily noticed.

Wound care post-operatively

- No dressing required for facial wound or sutures
- Wound care is vital with regular cleaning and removal of crusts and debris
- Regular application of chloramphenicol ointment to the suture line (a non-antibiotic ointment may also be used)
- Suture removal at 4 to 7 days depending upon site
- Explanation to the patient of the stages of wound healing will help them understand the slow improvement (Table 11.2)

Table 11.2 Phases of scar healing

- Red phase   – first 2 to 3 months. Red, raised, tight and itchy scar.
- Pink phase – slow settlement of scar over next few months.
- White phase – scar becomes pale, soft and flat, blends into facial lines. Complete at one year.

Skin grafts

Skin grafts may be the treatment of choice in certain defects, but equally may be the only option because of lack of adjacent tissue or size of defect. Full thickness skin grafts, harvested from the post-auricular area or the supraclavicular area of the neck, are suitable for facial reconstruction, particularly for certain nasal sites (Fig. 11.13(a), (b) and (c)), the lower eyelid, ear, temple or forehead. Some contraction occurs (but less than secondary intention healing), and this must be taken into consideration.

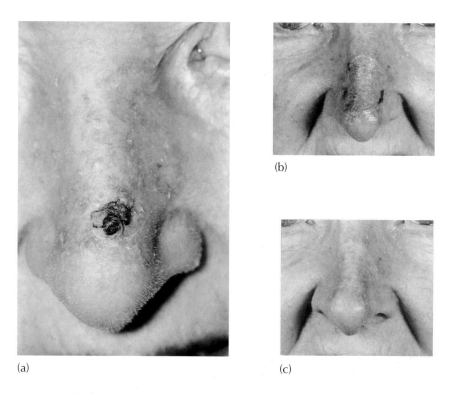

(a)   (b)   (c)

Fig. 11.13(a), (b) and (c)   Basal cell carcinoma of the nose, repaired with full thickness skin graft. (a) Pre-operative; (b) 3 weeks after surgery; (c) 3 months after surgery.

Split thickness skin grafts, harvested from the inner thigh with a manual or electric dermatome, are useful for scalp defects.

For all skin grafts there must be sufficient vascular tissue in the defect bed to support the graft, allowing initial diffusion of oxygen and nutrients to the graft followed by revascularisation of the graft by the fourth to seventh day. Bare bone, cartilage or tendon will not allow grafts to take and other reconstructive options must be employed. After grafting, avoidance of movement or shear in the healing phase is important, along with prevention of infection and haematoma, and usually a dressing such as a tie-over pack is used for 5 to 10 days.

Wound care post-operatively

- Post-operatively the patient is nursed sitting up, and procedures leading to significant elevation of blood pressure avoided.
- A Jelonet and proflavin wool tie-over pack is removed at 5 to 10 days depending on graft type.
- Peripheral and quilting sutures are carefully removed.
- Non-adherent dressings are used for the first week after suture removal, especially with split thickness grafts to the scalp, to prevent accidental movement or trauma.
- The daily removal of crusts from wounds is important.

Local flaps

Local tissue that can be moved into the surgical defect and still allow closure of the donor site can offer significant advantages in reconstruction:

- It can cover bare bone and cartilage
- Tissue bulk can be restored
- It avoids distortion
- It is aesthetically superior

Design of these flaps takes into account the natural facial lines, junction lines and relaxed skin tension lines and, where possible, places the resulting scars in these lines to achieve camouflage. This irregular pattern is often less noticeable than a long linear scar and flaps allow reconstruction with adjacent tissue of similar colour, texture and thickness. These advantages come with disadvantages for they require additional incisions and tissue movements, and may lead to increased complication risks and require greater surgical skill, knowledge and practice. It is important to:

- Consider the lesion and resulting defect
- Consider the patient

■ Consider the reconstructive options and involve the patient in an active discussion before reaching a final decision

The use of visual aids such as diagrams and before and after photographs of similar lesions showing progress of healing and maturation of scars over one year are very useful in counselling the patient and in developing their understanding and tolerance of the surgery and its likely reasonable functional and aesthetic result.

Wound care post-operatively

■ Suture line care as before.
■ Flaps placed into concavities, e.g. medial canthal area at side of nose, benefit from pressure dressings which mould them gently, without ischaemia, into the correct shape. Thermoplastic nasal splints will hold jelonet dressings effectively in these areas but they may require a fresh dressing on the first post-operative day.
■ The patient is nursed sitting up or with the head elevated post-operatively.
■ Sutures are removed at 5 to 7 days.

The concepts of facial cosmetic units and subunits, lines of relaxed skin tension and reservoirs of spare tissue are useful in reconstructive surgery. Cosmetic or aesthetic units such as the nose, eyelids, cheeks, temples, upper and lower lips are each areas with different skin characteristics. These units may be further divided into subunits.

The junction lines (Fig. 11.14) along with the visible wrinkle lines and lines seen in facial expression allow scar placement with maximum disguise, but skin tension lines are not usually visible and may not always coincide with the patient's visible lines. These lines indicate the directional pull that exists in relaxed skin and surgical incisions should parallel these lines.

Flap movement

Three classic movements of tissue in flaps are described.

■ Advancement   (Fig. 11.15(a) and (b))
■ Rotation   (Fig. 11.16(a), (b), (c) and (d))
■ Transposition   (Fig. 11.17(a), (b) and (c))

Frequently there are combinations of these movements. When tissue is moved from one site to another, as well as the primary movement (movement of the flap), secondary movement of adjacent tissue occurs on suturing, that is the flap pulls the tissue towards it. Care must taken if

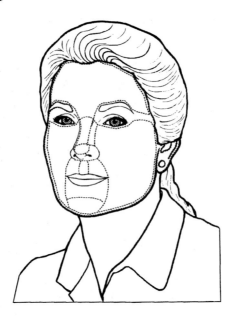

Fig. 11.14   Junction lines of the face.

close to free or distortable margins such as eyelids, lips or nasal rim, that this secondary movement does not spoil the repair.

Use of flaps on the face

Cheek

There is usually plentiful spare lax tissue and favourable lines in which to place incisions. The younger cheek, however, has fewer lines in which to hide and utilisation of relaxed skin tension lines is important.

The medial cheek, as it meets the nose, is a common site for BCCs and the subcutaneous based triangular advancement flap is frequently useful. This flap has the skin cut in a triangular fashion but its deep connections via the subcutaneous fat are intact and lax, so allowing advancement based on its subcutaneous pedicle. Careful closure in a V–Y fashion completes the reconstruction (Fig. 11.18(a), (b) and (c)).

Forehead

Advancement flaps which make maximal use of the horizontal creases and minimal use of the vertical incisions are favoured here (*see* Fig. 11.15(a), (b) and (c)).

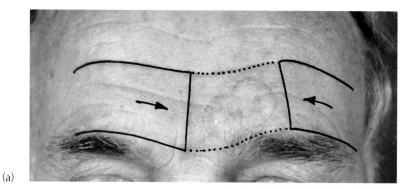

(a)

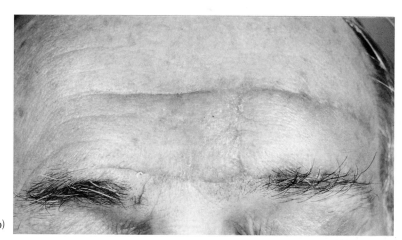

(b)

Fig. 11.15(a) and (b) Advancement flaps for reconstruction of defect following excision of basal cell carcinoma of forehead. (a) Outline of excision and flaps; (b) 2 weeks after surgery.

Temple

This is an area which often has sufficient spare tissue for local flaps such as the rhomboid design, but larger lesions may require skin grafting.

Nose

This is one of the most challenging areas of the face to reconstruct and a variety of flaps may be used according to the site and extent of the tumour and which cosmetic subunits are involved in the tumour and the prospective repair.

Bilobed flaps are frequently used (Fig. 11.19(a), (b) and (c)) to good effect, but dorsal nasal flaps are useful (Fig. 11.20(a), (b) and (c)), and two stage

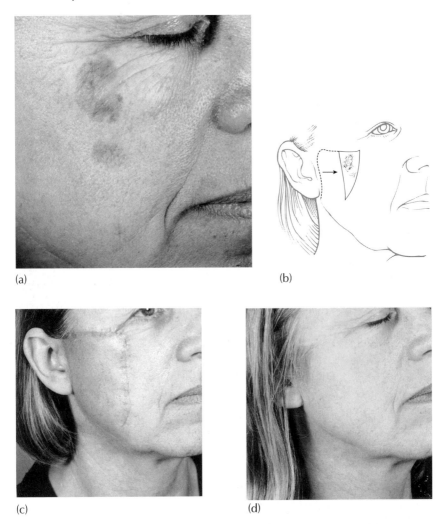

(a)   (b)

(c)   (d)

Fig. 11.16 (a), (b), (c) and (d)   Rotation flap of cheek following excision of lentigo maligna. (a) Pre-operative; (b) outline of excision and flap; (c) 2 weeks after surgery; (d) 6 months after surgery.

flaps from the naso-labial area or mid forehead allow reconstruction of larger or more complex skin cancers (Fig. 11.21(a), (b), (c) and (d)). In this technique a flap is raised and transposed to the defect, but jumps over normal tissue to get there. The mid portion is dressed to prevent adherence to normal skin and over 3–4 weeks the repair gains a blood supply from its new tissue bed. The flap is then divided and inset carefully at both origin and destination. The excess tissue in the middle is disposed of as the original donor site has been closed primarily or skin grafted. Cancers on

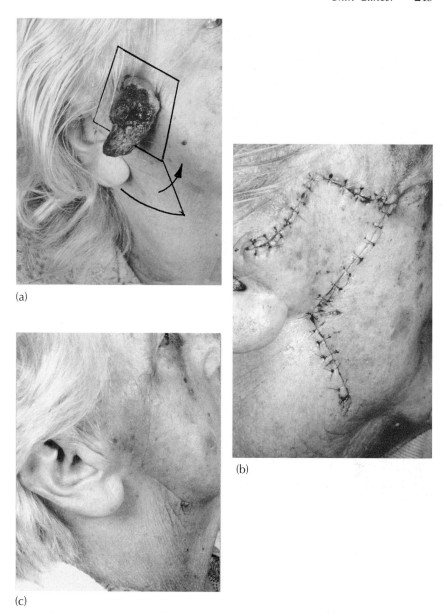

(a)

(b)

(c)

Fig. 11.17(a), (b) and (c) Transposition flap of cheek following excision of squamous cell carcinoma. (a) Outline of excision and flap; (b) flap transposed and sutured in place; (c) final result.

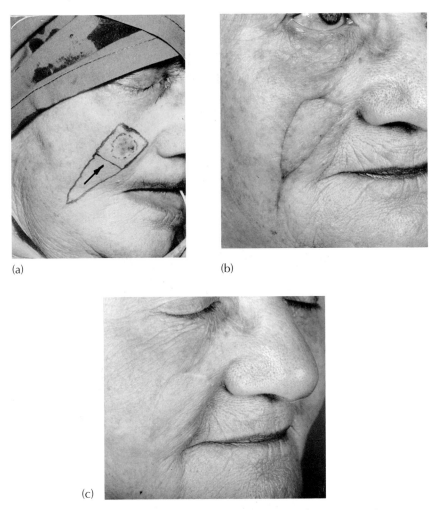

(a)

(b)

(c)

Fig. 11.18(a), (b) and (c)   Advancement cheek flap for repair of excision of squamous carcinoma. (a) At operation showing lines for flap and excision of tumour; (b) 2 weeks after surgery; (c) 6 months after surgery.

the bridge of the nose can encroach upon the medial aspect of the eyelids and careful excision, preserving the medial canthal tendon and the lachrymal apparatus, is required. Skin grafts or the simple transposition flaps from the glabella region (skin above the nasal bridge) work well.

Ear

Small to middle sized defects after tumour excision which do not involve the free margins of the ear are well constructed by full thickness skin

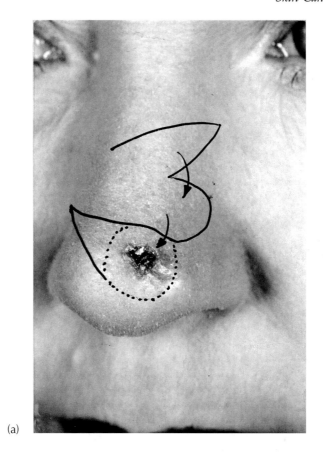

(a)

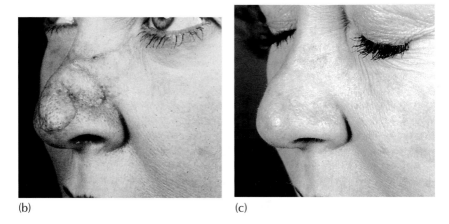

(b)   (c)

Fig. 11.19(a), (b) and (c)   Bilobed flap for repair of basal cell carcinoma of the nose. (a) Outline of flap; (b) 3 weeks after surgery; (c) 1 year after surgery.

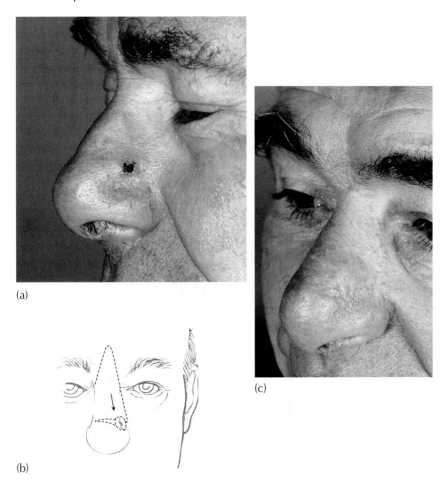

(a)

(b)

(c)

Fig. 11.20(a), (b) and (c)   Dorsal nasal flap to repair excision of nasal basal cell carcinoma. (a) Pre-operative; (b) outline for excision and rotation flap with back cut; (c) 6 months post-operative.

grafts. The underlying cartilage is taken with the excision, so allowing a graft to be placed onto the remaining skin. Contour is usually well maintained. Flaps are useful for larger reconstruction and the post-auricular area is a useful supply of skin. Preservation of somewhere to put the arm of spectacles is of great long term benefit to a patient. Some large tumours require amputation of the ear and its reconstruction, if desired, using natural tissue or via a prosthetic ear effectively retained by osseointegrated implants.

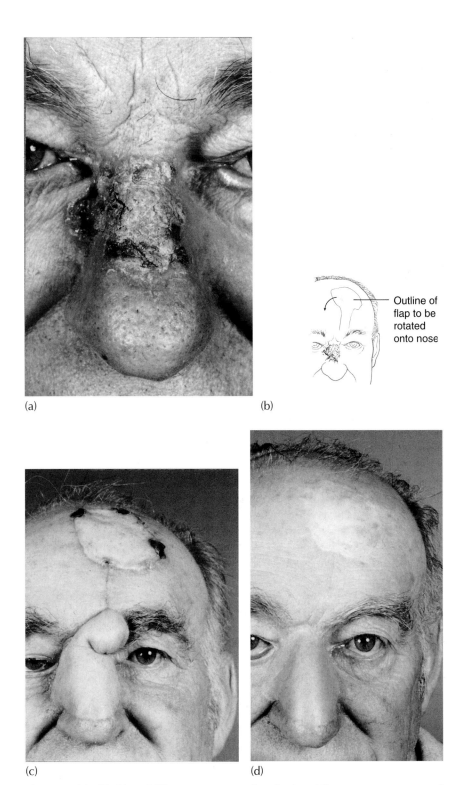

Outline of
flap to be
rotated
onto nose

(a)

(b)

(c)

(d)

Fig. 11.21(a), (b), (c) and (d) Two stage median forehead flap to repair excision of large nasal basal cell carcinoma. (a) Pre-operative; (b) outline of flap to be rotated onto nose after excision of tumour; (c) before second stage operation; (d) 8 months after initial operation.

11

Part III
The Role of the Head and Neck Nurse Specialist

L. Knighton

The development of the head and neck cancer specialist nurse

The value of a nurse with site specific skills and education has been well documented within the nursing literature for a number of years, although the head and neck cancer specialist is a relatively new phenomenon. The first post was established in the Cookridge Hospital in Leeds in 1991, with 3 years' funding from Macmillan Cancer Relief. Currently there are 12 such posts in Britain, all of which are hospital based, as well as many more which do not receive Macmillan funding, but which provide support and information for patients diagnosed with cancer of the head and neck area.

Such posts can be seen as a response to a number of factors:

- The Report of the Expert Advisory Group on Cancer (Calman-Hine 1995) which advocated the development of nurses with site specific expertise.
- The poor prognosis of head and neck cancer which has remained unchanged for the last 40 years.
- Developments in cancer treatments mean that patients are living longer following a diagnosis of cancer, hence a greater need for support and symptom control.
- The anatomical importance of structures affected, namely the aerodigestive tract and most of the vital senses.
- Psychosocial and economic problems associated with this patient group including old age, poverty, alcohol and tobacco dependence.

All Macmillan clinical nurse specialist post holders are first level registered nurses, educated to at least diploma level, with 5 years' clinical experience within the relevant clinical setting. For the head and neck cancer specialist nurse this may include the specialties of oral and maxillofacial surgery, ENT surgery, plastic surgery and oncology.

The aims and objectives of the service provided reflect the specific needs of the patient group and nurses use their specialist skills and knowledge to improve the care offered to patients. The nurse does not act as the direct care giver, but acts via the carers, using the main components of the clinical nurse specialist role:

- Education
- Research
- Consultation
- Expert nurse clinician

The particular needs of patients with head and neck cancer

Head and neck cancer has a relatively low incidence, accounting for only 2 to 3% of all cancers in the UK, but the devastating nature of the disease and its treatments mean that the involvement of a specialist nurse is highly desirable.

Head and neck cancer, perhaps more than any other, dramatically alters the most basic of daily functions and interactions, including speech, eating and swallowing, as well as producing the all too obvious changes in appearance.

Treatments for head and neck cancer are usually multimodality, requiring extensive, disfiguring and dysfunctioning surgery, followed by approximately 4 to 6 weeks of radiotherapy which in itself causes significant side effects such as mucositis, pain and long term xerostomia. All of these factors cause distress for the patients and challenges for the professionals caring for them.

Diagnosis

Bad news is defined as any information that drastically alters a person's view of their future for the worse, creating feelings of anxiety, fear, uncertainty and hopelessness. It is here that the Macmillan nurse plays a vital role in support and information giving. This means ensuring that the patient and their family have all the verbal and written information that they require initially, while remembering that the amount of information individual patients require is variable, and that they will retain only a proportion of the information given verbally. Further information can be given gradually, over subsequent meetings, which should include family members whenever possible.

There is a wide range of written material and support groups available nationally that may supplement local sources.

Treatment

Radiotherapy and surgery are the mainstays of treatment for head and neck cancer, both of which can cause significant problems in both the short and long term. A multidisciplinary approach is necessary to support patients during this time, liaising closely with relevant professionals such as speech and language therapists and dieticians and ensuring continuity of care through effective communication. The head and neck specialist nurse has the knowledge and experience to support and guide the direct carers, acting in a consultative and resource capacity. This may be achieved when offering direct advice, for example on symptom management, as well as through the development of policies and protocols that can be used by others involved in patient care.

The nurse can refer to other sources if necessary for the patient's well-being, and must ensure that the patient has access to professionals who are aware of the details of their diagnosis and treatment. This may include the district nurse, general practitioner or relevant hospital ward.

Follow-up care

Professional input is vital to ensure that patients recover physically, socially and emotionally following their treatment, and the value of good social support systems in rehabilitation is well documented. The head and neck Macmillan nurse ensures that the patient has access to the full range of services available, monitoring their effectiveness and identifying areas of concern. The Macmillan nurse must also ensure that family members are supported during this time, and care must be taken to include them in the decision making whenever possible.

Due to the relatively low incidence of the disease, healthcare professionals may often have little experience in caring for patients with head and neck cancer. Discharge may be complicated, for example if the patient has a tracheostomy, therefore close liaison with professionals is an important aspect of the role of the specialist nurse. This may necessitate joint home visits, provision of relevant written and verbal information, as well as teaching applicable to the needs of care givers, both professionals and family members.

Follow-up care is also particularly important in view of the high levels of recurrent disease and the possibility of the development of a second primary tumour in approximately 9% of patients. This is particularly true if patients continue to smoke, and drink heavily. If necessary, patients must be educated and encouraged to curtail these habits.

Palliation

Unfortunately some patients will not be cured of their cancer and here the head and neck Macmillan nurse is often in an excellent position to initiate palliative care services. Patients may experience a range of complex problems, some of which are unique to head and neck cancer. Commonly identified problems include pain, fungating wounds, aerodigestive obstruction and haemorrhage. The head and neck nurse specialist ensures carers are supported. This is achieved by acting in an educational and consultative role, joint visits, regular updates on the patient's development, both written and verbal, and by providing a link to the acute sector. Referral to other professionals with specialist palliative skills is important, for example hospice in-patient and out-patient care, palliative care nurse specialists and pain specialists. Support for the family during this time is vital, and this may be ongoing if a bereavement service is offered. Due to the nature of the disease, which tends to remain loco-regional rather than causing distant metastases, patients often remain well with high performance status until very late in their disease. This short terminal phase complicates palliative care, since patients are often reluctant to consider palliative services until they become more obviously terminal, when deterioration may happen rapidly.

One of the benefits of a Macmillan head and neck service is the involvement of the specialist nurse in the patient's care from diagnosis, and with this relationship already established before the patient becomes terminally ill, the Macmillan nurse can identify problems more readily and refer on when necessary.

Conclusion

The head and neck nurse specialist is a new phenomenon, but is linked to an increased recognition of the need for nurses with site specific skills. The nature of head and neck cancer, and its devastating effects on function and appearance, creates many complex problems for professionals caring for this group of patients. This is exacerbated by a number of factors including the relatively low incidence of this cancer, which means that professionals often have limited experience in dealing with the problems associated with this cancer. There is also an awareness that this cancer is linked to patients who may be psychosocially vulnerable because of their age, or because of a history of alcohol and tobacco dependence. All of these factors create an enormous challenge to the nurse, and require a multi-disciplinary approach to care. The head and neck Macmillan nurse is in an ideal position to co-ordinate the multidisciplinary teams, providing continuity of care and ensuring that the patient has full access to the wide range of services and support necessary.

The following organisations can provide useful information and support:

- **Bacup:** telephone 0800 181199 (freephone)
- **Cancerlink:** helpline 0800 132905
- **Macmillan Cancer Relief:** telephone 020 7351 7811

12

Pre-prosthetic Surgery

G.T. Cheney

This chapter describes problems encountered by denture wearers which have surgical solutions. The aim of surgery is to correct abnormalities which prevent normal wearing of dentures. Pre-prosthetic surgery is the surgical preparation of the mouth to receive dentures. A prosthesis is an artificial device made to replace a part of the body which has been lost following surgery or trauma, or is congenitally missing or deformed. The problems which prevent the comfortable wearing of dentures are:

- Bony irregularities, e.g. retained roots, sharp alveolar ridges, prominent mylohyoid ridges, tori and alveolar ridge atrophy
- Soft tissue problems, e.g. denture granuloma, fibroma, shallow sulcus and 'floppy ridges'

Bony problems

Many bony or hard tissue irregularities of the edentulous (toothless) denture-bearing parts of the mouth are quite obvious to the eye, but X-rays should be taken to ensure that there are no underlying problems, such as buried roots or teeth present prior to denture construction. An OPT film is a good screening X-ray for the jaws.

The removal of any pathology must take into account important related structures, particularly nerves. Nerve damage must be avoided at all costs. The sensory nerves to the lower lip (inferior alveolar nerves) run in a bony canal within the mandible, exiting at the mental foramina in the premolar regions. The lingual nerves, responsible for taste and sensation to the tongue, are closely related to the lingual aspects of the mandible in the molar regions. These nerves are vulnerable during mandibular surgery and loss of sensation in the lip or tongue is one of the most unpleasant complications of oral surgery (Fig. 12.1).

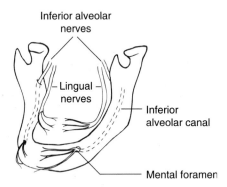

Fig. 12.1   The inferior alveolar and lingual nerves supplying the lower lip and tongue with sensation.

Sharp alveolar ridges

Some patients develop sharp bony prominences or irregularities following removal of their teeth. Much later, bony resorption of the ridges may produce a sharp 'knife edge' ridge. In either case pressure from the dentures on the bony spurs will cause pain and bone may need to be surgically smoothed to reduce discomfort (Fig. 12.2(a) and (b)) . However, if the denture is well made such surgery can often be avoided.

Mylohyoid ridges

These lie on the lingual side of the lower jaw in the molar regions and provide the attachment for the mylohyoid muscle which forms the floor

Fig. 12.2   Sharp lower alveolar ridge (a) before and (b) after smoothing.

of the mouth. In the edentulous patient the bony ridge and muscle can prevent a lower denture seating down comfortably or being extended properly, which will reduce its retention. The nipping of the mucosa between the denture and the sharp ridge can be the cause of considerable pain. A sharp mylohyoid ridge can be removed surgically giving relief and allowing the denture flange (the periphery or edge of the denture) to be fully extended into the lingual sulcus. This greatly improves the retention (Fig. 12.3).

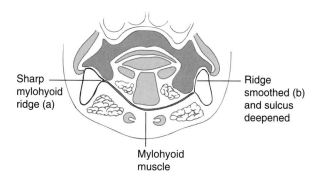

Fig. 12.3   Mylohyoid ridge (a) before and (b) after smoothing.

Tori

A torus is a spur or nodule of bone which can appear on the lingual side of the lower jaw in the premolar region (torus mandibularis, Fig. 12.4) and spoil the fit of a denture or cause soreness of the mucosa by nipping it between the bone and the denture flange. Similar bony growths or exostoses occur in the midline of the hard palate (torus palatinus, Fig. 12.5), but here they rarely interfere with the fit of an upper denture because they are on the posterior part of the bony palate. Problems can usually be avoided by designing the denture around them and not over them. However, the overlying mucosa can become sore by the constant trauma of mastication and this is a good reason to excise them.

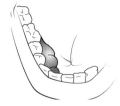

Fig. 12.4   Torus mandibularis

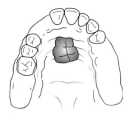

Fig. 12.5   Torus palatinus.

Ridge atrophy

Once alveolar bone has been lost either naturally or surgically, it cannot be replaced except by bone grafting or ridge augmenting procedures using material such as hydroxyapatite. Such procedures are complicated, time consuming and have an unpredictable outcome. They have largely been replaced by implant treatment (*see below*).

Soft tissue problems

The mucosa which lines the mouth is, for the main part, well designed to withstand the constant wear and tear of chewing food. The surfaces chiefly involved in mastication are those of the tongue (the dorsum) and the palate. Here the mucosa is thickened and very tough, well designed to play its role in chewing. Nevertheless trauma, usually from the teeth or dentures, can cause damage in the form of ulceration. This can normally be dealt with by smoothing down sharp teeth or an overextended denture flange, which quickly relieves the discomfort.

Denture granuloma (fibroma, hypertrophy, hyperplasia)
(*see also* Chapter 6)

Ill fitting dentures, especially if worn at night as well as during the day, produce less severe trauma causing low grade chronic inflammation of the mucosa leading to hypertrophy around the periphery or flange of the denture (denture granuloma, Fig. 12.6). Surprisingly the condition often goes unnoticed by the patient, although the excess mucosa may interfere with the fit of a denture, attract infections such as thrush, lead to acute inflammation or occasionally develop a neoplastic appearance.

Treatment is normally undertaken under local anaesthetic in the out-patient department. The hypertrophic mucosa is excised, leaving intact the underlying tissue covering the bone. This leaves a raw area (which usually heals rapidly), but no attempt is made to close the wound by suturing, as this will decrease the sulcus depth. The dentures are usually

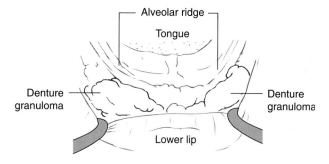

Fig. 12.6 Denture granuloma caused by ill fitting lower denture.

relined immediately post-operatively with a lining of tissue conditioner. This protects the wound during healing, controls bleeding, retains the depth of the sulcus and, most importantly, gives back the patient their appearance and ability to chew. Once healing has occurred, new dentures can be made.

The removal of mucosal hypertrophy at the posterior border of the hard palate leaves a wound which cannot normally be sutured. Although the excess tissue can be cut using a scalpel, it can also be despatched by diathermy (high frequency electrical cutting), leaving a smaller wound which heals rapidly without the need for protective covering.

Occasionally, skin grafting may be necessary following the excision of very extensive denture hypertrophy (*see below* vestibuloplasty).

Most soft tissue problems can be avoided by good denture hygiene and regular checking of dentures for fit. All patients should be advised to remove their dentures last thing at night, to clean them thoroughly under lukewarm water with a soft brush and to soak them in a proprietary brand of denture cleaner. If they are worn by day and night mucosal lesions are more likely to occur and patients are also prone to Candida infection ('thrush').

Leaf fibroma (Fig. 12.7)

A specific type of hypertrophy can occur in the palate beneath an upper denture. The hypertrophic tissue is localised and flattened and attached by a narrow stalk which behaves like a hinge allowing the lesion to fold downwards – a leaf fibroma. Removal is by excision of the base of the stalk which tends to bleed briskly as it carries the blood vessels to the lesion. This can be controlled by temporarily relining the denture and refitting it immediately.

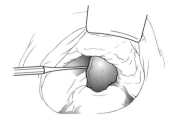

Fig. 12.7 Leaf fibroma.

Shallow sulcus

The denture-bearing bony ridges of the jaws gradually resorb and atrophy with age. This leads to the loss of depth of the sulcus and poor denture retention. It is sometimes possible to recover the sulcus by a deepening procedure (vestibuloplasty). This is achieved by either inserting a skin graft in the lower labial sulcus or by undermining the muscle attachments in the upper labial sulcus. The skin for the former is taken from the inside of the upper arm or thigh and inlaid into the prepared oral wound, supporting it with a splint or modified denture firmly fixed in place by wires or strong sutures passed around the jaw. When the splint is removed after 10 to 14 days the graft has normally taken well, but as the wound heals the graft tends to shrink, reducing the depth of the newly acquired sulcus. This can be controlled to some extent by fitting a new denture with well extended flanges as soon as the splint is removed. In spite of this, much of the new sulcus may be lost over the ensuing year. For this reason vestibuloplasty has been overtaken by the use of implants (*see below*).

The technique in the upper jaw is more successful. Once the muscle attachments underlying the mucosa have been released, there is an immediate increase in sulcus depth which is then maintained by inserting the new extended denture and holding it in place with small bone screws inserted through the denture into the alveolar bone. The screws are removed at 10 to 14 days and the denture cleaned, temporarily lined with conditioner and reinserted. This is one of the few occasions that a patient is allowed to wear the denture 24 hours a day, but only for a prescribed period (Fig. 12.8).

Fibrous (floppy) ridges

Sometimes the alveolar bone forming the ridge will resorb more rapidly than usual and be replaced by fibrous tissue creating a floppy ridge, giving indifferent support for the denture. This is most commonly seen in the anterior part of the upper jaw when natural lower teeth bite against the upper denture, producing high forces which cause ridge resorption.

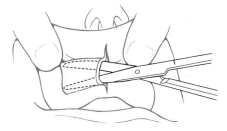

Fig. 12.8 Undermining and detachment of mucosal attachments in maxillary vestibuloplasty.

Floppy ridges can be improved by excising some of the unsupported soft tissue, but there is a risk of leaving insufficient ridge to retain a denture (Fig. 12.9(a), (b) and (c)). Again, a well designed denture can usually be provided without the need to resort to surgery.

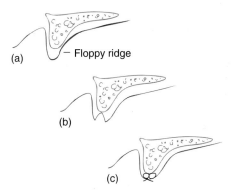

Fig. 12.9 (a) Floppy ridge in anterior maxilla (cross sectional sagittal view); (b) simple wedge excision of redundant tissue; (c) closure.

Frenectomy (*see also* Chapter 6)

A frenum is a band of mucosa arising from the soft tissues of the sulcus and attached close to the crest of the bony ridge (Fig. 12.10). It can interfere with denture retention by upsetting the peripheral seal formed by the flange and for this reason it may need to be removed. In patients with natural teeth such bands may cause the formation of a diastemma or gap between the central maxillary incisors. The removal of a mucosal frenum, a frenectomy, will often improve the fit and retention of a denture.

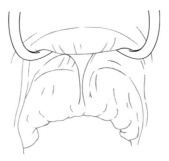

Fig. 12.10   Upper labial frenum.

Implants

Intra-oral implants

The arrival of reliable implant systems has revolutionised preprosthetic surgery, making redundant many of the surgical techniques to increase the bony ridges by bone grafting and sulcus deepening by skin grafting. However, some minor surgical procedures will always be required to deal with buried roots and teeth, local pathology and soft tissue problems. There may also be the need to improve the support for an implant by grafting bone to augment the ridge, but the larger procedures are in the main no longer necessary.

Implants ('fixtures') are screw-like cylinders made of titanium and are literally screwed into the alveolar bone after careful surgical preparation. The implant is left in place for 3 to 5 months as a first stage to allow it to become 'osseointegrated'. While some doubt that true integration of the metal with surrounding bone occurs, there is no doubt that once the implant has 'taken', it is virtually impossible to remove. In addition, to prevent infection, a good soft tissue seal is essential around the neck of the implant where it penetrates the mucosa.

The success of the implant depends on several factors:

- The surgical care taken at insertion
- The skill of the prosthodontist and maxillofacial technician who plan the position of implants and make and fit the final prosthesis
- Patients must be highly motivated and able to maintain a high standard of oral hygiene for the long term success of implants

Described in this section is the use of implants to aid retention of dentures, but implants are also used for single tooth replacement and as supports for fixed bridgework in the mouth.

The first stage

This is carried out under full sterile conditions in the clinic or operating theatre. It may be a lengthy procedure and the patient is frequently offered sedation if it is to be performed under local anaesthesia. After the fixtures have been inserted, the soft tissue wound is closed completely and the denture, suitably adjusted to prevent trauma, may be worn after initial healing has taken place.

The second stage

This takes place after 3 months for mandibular implants and 5 months for those in the maxilla. It is a relatively short procedure and entails the uncovering of the top of the fixture and its cover screw by removal of a round plug of overlying mucosa. The cover screws are removed and replaced by abutments which screw firmly into the end of the fixture and protrude through the mucosa just above the level of the gingiva. The denture then requires modification to allow it to be worn again until the final prosthesis is ready for insertion, usually only a matter of a few weeks.

Some systems use a single stage procedure leaving the implants exposed, rather than covered at the first stage as described above. However, the same interval is still required (3 to 5 months) for osseointegration to occur before construction of the final prosthesis can take place.

The stages and principles involved in implant placement and prosthetic reconstruction are essentially similar wherever the site. The example described here is for implant placement in the anterior region of the lower jaw as an aid to the support and retention of a lower denture. Atrophy of the ridge has made normal wearing of the denture difficult or impossible.

Indications

Inability to wear lower denture.

Aims

Restoration of function and appearance.

Pre-operative preparation of the patient

- A full discussion of what is involved and the likely outcome, with special reference to the long term care of implants (Information leaflet No 13)
- Informed consent
- If for general anaesthetic, complete standard check list

PATIENT INFORMATION LEAFLET No 13

ORAL and MAXILLOFACIAL SURGERY DEPARTMENT

IMPLANTS

1. Implants are titanium cylinders which are screwed into the jaws to replace the roots of natural teeth which have been lost. An average implant would be 12 mm long and 4 mm wide. They may be used singly or in groups.
2. The implants are then used to carry crowns or bridges, or to stabilise dentures which are constructed separately.
3. Initially an examination is carried out to determine the patient's suitability for implants and to plan any intended procedure. Models and X-rays are necessary for this.
4. The procedure may be carried out under local or general an anaesthesia. An incision is made in the gum and the bone carefully drilled to hold the implant. The implant can then be inserted.
5. The implant must now be allowed to heal into the bone for about 3 months. After this the crown, bridge or denture is constructed to fit onto the implant or implants.
6. Between 5% and 10% of implants fail and need to be removed. The most important factor in the long term success of implants is the day-to-day care which patients must provide for themselves. **Oral hygiene must be scrupulous.** Methodical and thorough cleaning must take place around each implant on a twice daily basis using methods which are usually similar to normal tooth brushing and flossing.
7. If oral hygiene is not of the highest order, the implants will fail.

Procedure

Prior to surgery, detailed planning will have taken place. This would include radiographs and models and the construction of surgical templates as an aid to the placement of the implant.

Instruments required

- Oral surgical set (*see* Fig. 4.5)
- Low speed drill with irrigation
- Intra-oral implantation instruments and implants

Anaesthesia

Local or general.

Positioning

Standard for clinic or operating theatre.

Preparation

Standard peri-oral.

Operative procedure (Fig. 12.11)

- A mucoperiosteal flap is raised to expose the surgical field.
- The ridge, if sharp or irregular, may need to be smoothed with a large bone bur to create a flat surface of sufficient width.
- The position of the implants is marked on the bone with a small round bur, using a surgical template if necessary.
- Each implant site is prepared to the predetermined depth using drills of increasing diameter to gradually widen the site. All drilling is carried out at low speed using intermittent pressure and profuse irrigation.
- After the depth of the preparation has been checked a thread is tapped into the implant site.
- The implant is screwed into the site and a cover screw fixed onto the implant.
- Some systems close the wound completely at this stage, others close around the implants which project just through the mucosa.
- If the procedure is carried out in two stages, the second stage (at 3 to 5 months) involves making a small incision to confirm the position of the implant and removing a disc of tissue to uncover the implant.

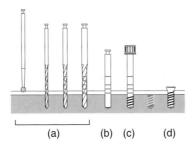

Fig. 12.11   Diagram to show steps carried out in implant placement. (a) Drilling; (b) measuring; (c) tapping; (d) implant placement.

Post-operative care and follow up

- Standard written post-operative instructions
- Antibiotics (for the first stage) and analgesics are prescribed
- Oral hygiene instruction
- A review appointment at one week

Complications

- Wound infection
- Damage to adjacent structures e.g. teeth and nerves. In the mandible the inferior alveolar nerve is at risk in its canal or at the mental foramen

The final stage (prosthodontic)

This involves taking impressions of the abutments and surrounding bony ridge so that the final prosthesis can be constructed. In this instance the prosthesis must be removable to allow the implants to be kept clean and healthy and several methods of attachment are available. In the case illustrated the prosthesis (lower denture) simply clips onto ball-ended attachments (abutments) screwed into the implants (Figs. 12.12 and 12.13).

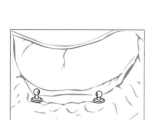

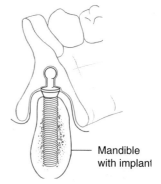

Mandible
with implant

Fig. 12.12 Implants with ball-ended attachments.

Fig. 12.13 Diagram with lower denture sectioned to show relationship with implant.

The implants and abutments must be cared for by the patient in exactly the same way as the natural teeth should have been, with regular oral hygiene (brushing and flossing) and periodic checks by the clinician. The abutments will need to be scaled, with nylon not metal instruments to prevent damage to the titanium surfaces, and carefully polished. Every 2 to 3 years implant supported bridges should be removed for close inspection and cleaning by the laboratory.

Although implant treatment is expensive in terms of the cost of the materials and clinician's time, the results are always rewarding, more so since there is every prospect of the treatment lasting many years, especially if it is well maintained.

Extra-oral implants

Extra-oral implants followed the successful use of jaw implants and the principles of placement are identical. The implants are shorter (3 to 4 mm) and have a flange for stability. The skin surrounding the implant is deliberately thinned so that it attaches firmly to the underlying bone, providing a good seal at the skin–implant interface.

Implants can be used to support facial prostheses replacing tissue which has been lost either through the ravages of cancer and its treatment, as the result of trauma or is congenitally missing. Most commonly involved are:

- Ears
- Eyes
- Noses

Larger prostheses masking the loss of facial tissue and the underlying bone of the maxilla can be supported by implants which in turn provide good anchorage for dentures as well as artificial eyes and noses. The twin aims of all facial and oral prostheses are the restoration of function and appearance. Implants are also used for the attachment of bone anchored hearing aids.

Implant placement in the temporal bone will be described, to provide attachment for a congenitally missing ear.

Pre-operative preparation of the patient

- Full discussion of the procedure with the patient (and parents if appropriate) with special reference to the long term care of the implant sites
- Informed consent
- The hair should be washed thoroughly the night before surgery
- The hair line is shaved approximately 5 cm beyond the operation site

Procedure

Instruments required

- Extra-oral tissue set
- Low speed drill with torque control and irrigation

- Extra-oral implantation instruments and implants
- Skin grafting instruments
- Local anaesthetic (2% lignocaine with 1 in 200 000 adrenaline)

Anaesthesia

General with orotracheal intubation.

Positioning

Standard with slight head uptilt and the head rotated to the opposite side.

Preparation

- Standard skin preparation
- Standard drapes with head towels to expose the operative site

Operative procedure

- The implant sites are tattooed with marking ink and an effort made to mark the bone with ink at these points. Ideal sites are 2 cm behind the ear canal opening at approximately 8 o'clock and 11 o'clock (on the right side) (Fig. 12.14).
- The skin is infiltrated with local anaesthetic.
- A curved incision is made 2 to 3 cm behind the implant site, and the skin and subcutaneous tissue reflected forwards.
- The periosteum is incised and reflected to expose the bone previously marked.
- Shouldered round burs to limit penetration are used to drill the

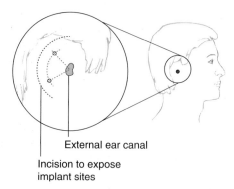

External ear canal

Incision to expose
implant sites

Fig. 12.14 Right post-auricular region showing ideal implant sites at 11 o'clock and 8 o'clock.

pilot holes (Fig. 12.15), followed by countersink drills to a depth of either 3 or 4 mm depending on the depth of bone available (Fig. 12.16).

- The implant site is tapped. All drilling and tapping is carried out at low speed and with profuse irrigation.
- The implant is screwed into position (Fig. 12.17). After placement of a cover screw, the incision is closed if the procedure has been planned for two stages and a pressure dressing applied.

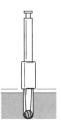

Fig. 12.15   Pilot hole drilled with shouldered bur.

Fig. 12.16   Countersink drilling.

Fig. 12.17   Implant screwed into position with cover screw ready for insertion.

If the procedure is being carried out in one stage, or 3 months later as a second stage procedure:

- The skin surrounding the implants is thinned and perforated (using a biopsy punch) at each implant site. Alternatively, the skin surrounding the implants can be excised and replaced by full or partial thickness skin grafts which are perforated in the same way. Whichever method is used the aim is to produce an area of thin hairless skin around the implants which is immobile and provides a good seal at the skin–implant interface.
- Abutment cylinders are fixed to the implants and plastic caps attached to each abutment. The healing caps allow a ribbon gauze dressing carrying an antibiotic ointment to be wound around the implants applying pressure to the flap or skin graft and preventing haematoma formation.
- A standard 'mastoid' pressure dressing is applied to complete the procedure.

Post-operative care and follow-up

- The pressure dressing is removed 24 to 48 hours after surgery.
- One week after surgery the healing caps and ribbon gauze dressing are removed and the area cleaned and redressed in the same way for a further week.
- After this the area may be left uncovered and cleaned gently by the patient with soap and water.
- One month after completion of the second stage of the procedure (or 3 to 4 months if the procedure is carried out in a single stage), the maxillofacial technician commences construction of the ear prosthesis. This involves taking impressions of the implant abutments followed by a long and complicated laboratory process involving considerable skill and artistry. The finished silicone prosthesis usually clips onto a bar spanning the abutments (Fig. 12.18).
- A regular daily cleaning routine must be established by (or for) the patient. Implants which are not scrupulously looked after will become crusted and infected and eventually fail.
- Once a stable healing condition has been reached a 6 month follow-up is adequate.

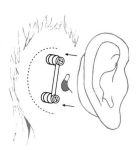

Fig. 12.18   Implants with connecting bar ready to receive prosthetic ear.

Complications

Inflammation and infection around the implants has several causes:

- Poor hygiene
- Skin which is too thick, and therefore mobile, creating a poor seal at the skin–implant interface
- Loose abutments

Summary

Many patients rely on dentures to restore oral function and facial aesthetics. Difficulties with the fit and comfort of dental prostheses may produce a serious handicap for some patients. A wide variety of surgical procedures is available to correct a range of problems. Relatively recently, endosseous implants have been developed which greatly improve the retention and stability of both intra-oral and extra-oral prostheses.

13

Cleft Lip and Palate

G. Pell

This chapter describes the surgical treatment of the cleft lip and palate patient. Primary surgery is carried out at relatively few centres and is covered here in outline only. Secondary surgery is practised more widely and is therefore covered in more detail. The aim of all surgery is to restore normal function (and aesthetics) with minimal impairment to growth and development of the upper jaw. The management of the cleft baby is a complex and prolonged task in patient care. It involves the combined skills of a number of professionals with expertise in this work, and may extend from birth to 20 years of age.

Classification

The incidence of all types of cleft lip and palate is 1 in 600 births. The anatomical site of the cleft usually classifies the different types of cleft.

Cleft lip

The incidence of a cleft lip only is about 25% of all cases. These clefts may be right or left sided, and may vary from a small notch in the lip to a fully developed cleft involving the lip and the alveolus but not the palate (Fig. 13.1).

Unilateral cleft lip and palate

The unilateral cleft may be either right or left sided, and involves the lip and hard and soft palates. This cleft divides the palate into a major seg-

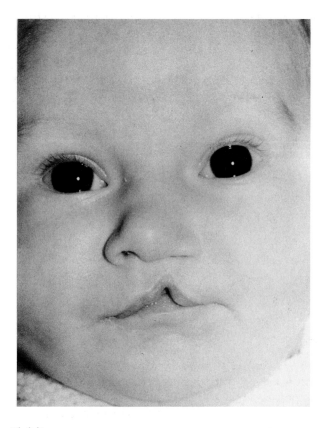

Fig. 13.1 Cleft lip.

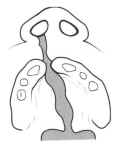

Fig. 13.2 Unilateral cleft lip and palate.

ment, which includes the premaxilla, and a minor segment. The incidence of a unilateral cleft lip and palate accounts for about 40% of all cases (Fig. 13.2).

Bilateral cleft lip and palate

The bilateral cleft separates the premaxilla from the rest of the palate, which itself has a cleft running along its length. The palate is therefore in three segments – the anteriorly placed premaxilla and the two lateral maxillary segments. The premaxilla has developing within it the central and lateral incisors, which tend to be crowded and short of space for normal development. Ten per cent of all clefts are bilateral (Fig. 13.3).

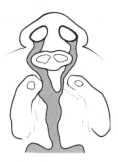

Fig;. 13.3 Bilateral cleft lip and palate.

Cleft palate

In this group, the lip and alveolus is not affected, but the cleft involves the hard and soft palates only to a varying degree. In some cases a submucous cleft may be present in the soft palate, and is due to the presence of a cleft in the muscle layer in the soft palate. Clefts of the palate alone account for 25% of all cleft cases (Fig. 13.4).

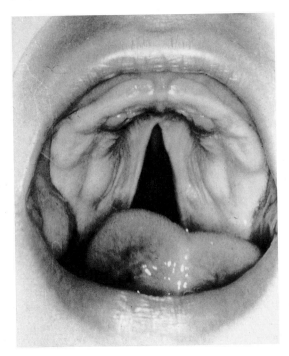

Fig. 13.4   Cleft palate.

Primary surgery

Primary surgery includes the repair of the lip and hard and soft palate. Clefts of the lip tend to be treated within 24 hours of birth, but there is a wide range among cleft palate teams as to when the palate should be treated. The advantage of repairing the lip early is to allow for easier feeding and improved aesthetics, while a delay for the palate repair will give the child a chance to become stronger, for further operations. Some surgeons will wait for 12 months before attempting to repair the hard and soft palates. There are a number of different techniques to repair the hard palate, which involve the stripping of the periosteum from the palatal bones. Although these procedures will result in the closure of the palatal cleft, secondary deformities develop, associated with the teeth, alveolus and the further growth of the jaws, due to the contraction of the scar tissue at the repaired cleft sites.

Secondary surgery

Secondary surgery involves operations on the facial cleft areas after a varying period of time has elapsed following the primary surgery. During growth of the face and jaws discrepancies will become apparent in both the hard and soft tissues which will require correction or revision. These include:

- The alveolar defect
- The lip and nose
- The soft palate and pharynx
- The jaws

The timing of these revisions varies with different cleft teams but it is usual to correct the bony tissues first, and deal with the soft tissues later. The orthodontist plays a key part in the treatment of the child, and is the appropriate clinician to take the lead and co-ordinate and monitor the future management of the child.

Alveolar defect

As a result of the discontinuity of the bone of the dental arch (alveolus) and nasal floor at the site of the cleft, a communication exists between the mouth and nose (oronasal fistula, Fig. 13.5). The discontinuity will result in:

- Leakage of fluids between mouth and nose.
- Collapse of the dental arches. In unilateral clefts the lesser segment collapses towards the midline. In bilateral clefts both lateral segments collapse behind the premaxilla, accentuating and deforming the alveolar defect.
- Teeth in the vicinity of the cleft (lateral incisors and canines) will fail to erupt or erupt into the cleft itself. Restoration of the alveolar defect is carried out at 7 to 8 years and may involve pre-surgical orthodontic treatment followed by surgery to place an alveolar bone graft and close the fistula.

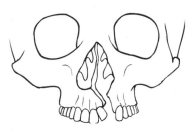

Fig. 13.5   The bony defect of the alveolus and nasal floor.

Pre-surgical orthodontics

Prior to any surgery for the correction of the alveolar defect, the orthodontist may re-expand the collapsed segments at about 7 to 8 years with fixed appliances. Any palatal fistulae present will increase with this palatal expansion, but it is easier to repair these defects after the maxillary expansion is complete. This phase of treatment may take up to 9 months.

Alveolar bone graft

Aims

■ Restoration of the continuity of the dental arch, thus stabilising the lesser segment, or in bilateral cases the premaxilla.

■ Closure of the oro-nasal fistula.

■ Provision of bone into which teeth can erupt naturally or be moved orthodontically. The teeth developing in the premaxilla and the lateral segments adjacent to the cleft are the lateral incisors and the canines. These important teeth are surrounded by scar tissue from previous surgery and cannot erupt normally. For a tooth to erupt into the mouth it must have cancellous bone surrounding it, and the tooth should be at the stage of its greatest eruptive potential (for lateral incisors and canines, about 7 to 8 years of age). In addition the mucosa overlying the bone at the site of tooth eruption must be keratinised so that healthy gingivae (gums) are formed. Any operation designed to enable teeth to erupt normally must therefore satisfy the above conditions. The cancellous bone is harvested from the upper end of the tibia or from the iliac crest.

Pre-operative preparation of the patient

Clinic

Following the completion of the orthodontics, and with the patient wearing a retaining appliance to prevent collapse of the dental arches, pre-operative X-rays of the alveolar cleft are taken. This is to evaluate the permanent teeth that are present, identify any supernumerary teeth that might need to be removed from the vicinity of the cleft and assess the eruptive state of the buried teeth.

Ward

The child may be admitted to the ward the day before the operation, and early contact is made with the patient and the parents and an opportunity given for any final questions to be answered. (Informed consent will usually have been given by the parents at the pre-assessment clinic.) The donor site and side for the bone graft is decided, and a mild sedative may be prescribed to allow a good night's sleep. The patient is usually first on the operating list, and after a suitable period of fasting, the child and parents come to the operating theatre.

Operating theatre procedure

Instruments required

- Intra-oral set (*see* Fig. 4.5)
- Extra-oral set with instruments for taking the bone graft (including trephine, osteotomes and gouges)

Anaesthesia

Nasotracheal intubation, if possible through the normal side of the nose.

Positioning

- Standard with a sand bag under the shoulders, and neck extended.
- If bone is to be taken from the tibia a sandbag is placed under the knee, and under the hip for iliac crest bone.

Preparation of operative site

It is important that during the skin preparation phase, the mouth and skin (donor) sites are prepared separately, to avoid contamination of the tibia or hip areas from the mouth.

Donor site
Standard skin preparation and towelling with sterile adhesive drape.

Mouth

- Standard perioral
- Standard head towels and drapes

Operative procedure

Donor site
Tibia and hip: the only bone that is placed into the cleft site is 'mushy' cancellous bone. Cartilage or cortical bone is not acceptable, as teeth can only erupt through the softer cancellous bone. The procedure therefore

entails removing the outer layer of cortical plate or cartilage from either site, until the cancellous bone is reached. Careful trephining and scooping of a sufficient quantity of this bone is performed. This bone is stored in saline and the donor site closed following haemostasis. Taking the bone graft can be delayed until the cleft has been completely prepared to receive the graft, shortening the time during which the viability of the graft may be reduced. Donor site pain can be reduced by the use of local anaesthetic delivered to the wound by a suitably placed cannula for the first 24 hours post-operatively.

The alveolus
- A small piece of mucosal scar tissue present in the notched area of the cleft is removed.
- Mucoperiosteal flaps are elevated adjacent to this defect and the bony margins of the whole cleft gradually exposed (Figs 13.6 and 13.7).
- Any scar tissue present within the cleft is removed, although it is important to preserve healthy mucoperiosteum or mucoperichondrium which will form the palatal and nasal layers of the repair.
- After closure of the nasal and palatal layers, the cancellous bone graft is placed into the space between the ends of the premaxillary and lateral bony segments, from the nasal to the oral mucosa, and compressed as tightly as possible.
- The buccal mucoperiosteal flap, that was elevated initially, is advanced (by incising the periosteum only) to cover the bone graft. Closure must be watertight, but not under tension. Synthetic resorbable sutures are normally used.

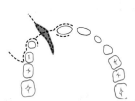
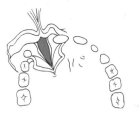

Fig. 13.6 Incision lines for exposure of alveolar cleft.   **Fig. 13.7** Flaps raised to expose bony cleft.

Post-operative care

Recovery is usually rapid and parents should be available to greet their child, either in the recovery area or after transfer to the ward. Surprisingly, post-operative pain is often greater from the donor site than from the oral region. The pain from the tibial site is generally slightly less than if bone had been taken from the hip.

- Antibiotics are given routinely, initially intravenously
- There is a strict 'nil by mouth' rule for the first 24 hours, followed by a 'clear fluids only' regime for the next 24 hours
- Oral hygiene is most important and chlorhexidine mouth baths are used every 4 hours
- After 48 hours, the patient can go on to a light diet, gradually resuming a normal diet in 3 to 4 days
- The patient is fit for discharge 3 to 5 days after the operation
- An out-patient appointment is given for one week later

Follow-up

- Skin sutures (donor site) are removed 10 days after surgery.
- If non-resorbable oral sutures are used, they are usually left in for 2 weeks.
- Post-operative X-rays are taken at 3 months to assess the volume and density of bone graft in the cleft.
- The patient is reviewed on the joint maxillofacial/orthodontic clinics at 3 monthly intervals and the eruption of any buried teeth in the cleft area is monitored.

Complications

- **Infection:** this is uncommon, but small spicules of bone may occasionally be shed into the mouth from the operation site. It is rare for large portions of the graft to be lost.
- **Pain:** pain from the hip with a characteristic limp (Trendelenberg gait) can be a problem, especially if an open, rather than a trephine technique, is used. Complications from a tibial site are few and a limp is uncommon.

Lip and nose

Secondary procedures on the lip and nose are best left until the alveolar bone graft has been completed and the tissues have settled. The support the premaxilla gives to the soft tissues is not easy to judge, and it is better to proceed slowly rather than promising results that may not be easy to attain.

Soft palate and pharynx

Poor speech in cleft patients is caused by a failure of the valve mechanism between the soft palate and pharynx (velopharyngeal incompetence). Secondary surgery on these structures (most commonly a pharyngoplasty) may be considered in some patients.

Jaws

Abnormalities of jaw growth arise as a result of previous primary surgery and the underlying tissue deficiency. The maxilla is mainly affected and in all three dimensions. This can result in a small retrusive maxilla and an elongated pseudo-prognathic mandible, giving a characteristic facial appearance (Fig. 13.8).

Correction of these major skeletal discrepancies is by osteotomy which cannot be considered until growth has ceased in the mid to late teens. Prior to surgery, orthodontic treatment aligns the teeth and dental arches to give the best dental occlusion after the osteotomy. The aim of the osteotomy is to advance the maxilla and often set back the mandible into a predetermined jaw relationship, which will give a good dental occlusion and a pleasing, balanced profile (Fig. 13.9). The procedures used are those discussed in Chapter 7.

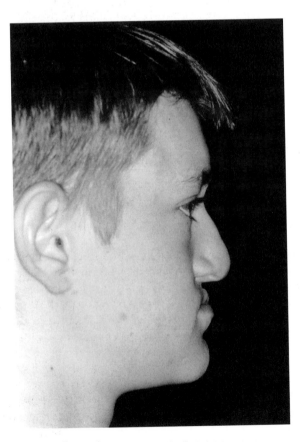

Fig. 13.8   Before maxillary advancement osteotomy.

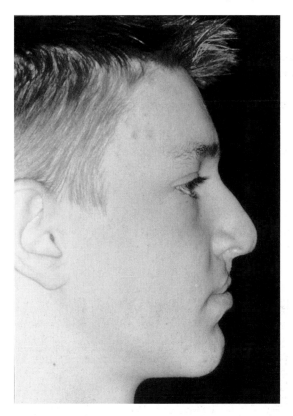

Fig. 13.9 After maxillary advancement osteotomy.

Summary

Although emphasis in this chapter is on the surgical aspects of the treatment of the cleft deformity, it must be further emphasised that a multidisciplinary team is involved at all stages. In addition to surgeons this would include an orthodontist, a paediatrician and a speech and language therapist. Also, counselling services must be available to parents from an early stage and support groups have a valuable role to play.

The total care of a cleft patient requires a great deal of time and expertise. Treatment may last for over 20 years, but if the result is a patient who is well integrated into society and has a pleasing and harmonious facial appearance, then the effort will have been well worthwhile.

Suggested further reading

The Calman Hine Report (1995) Report of an Expert Advisory Group on Cancer, HMSO, London.

Cawson, R.A. & Odell, E.W. (1999) *Oral Pathology: Colour Guide*, 2nd edn, Churchill Livingstone, Edinburgh.

Griffiths, J. & Boyle, S. (1993) *Colour Guide to Holistic Oral Care: a practical approach*, Mosby – Year Book, London.

Harris, M. & Reynolds, I.R. (1991) *Fundamentals of Orthognathic Surgery*, W.B. Saunders & Company.

Langdon, J.D. & Patel, M.F. (eds) (1998) *Operative Maxillofacial Surgery*, Chapman and Hall, London.

Loeb, S. (ed.) (1992) *Nursing Process in Clinical Practice*, Springhouse Corporation, Pennsylvania.

Mallett, J.M. & Bailey, C. (eds) (1998) *Royal Marsden NHS Trust Manual of Clinical Nursing Procedures*, 4th edn, Blackwell Science, Oxford.

HMSO (1994) *The Patients Charter, 1991* (updated 1994), HMSO, London.

Roper, N., Logan, W.W. & Tierney, A.J. (1996) *The Elements of Nursing*, 4th edn, Churchill Livingstone, Edinburgh.

Seward, G.R., Harris, M. & McGowan, D.A. (1987) *Outline of Oral Surgery*, Wright, Bristol.

Ward-Booth, P., Schendel, S.A. & Hausman, J. (eds) (1999) *Maxillofacial Surgery*, Churchill Livingstone, Edinburgh.

Williams, J.L.I. (ed.) (1994) *Rowe & Williams' Maxillofacial Injuries*, 2nd edn, Churchill Livingstone, Edinburgh.

Index